MICMAC
MEDICINES
Remedies and Recollections
■ ■ ■ ■ ■ ■ ■ ■ ■ ■ ■
Laurie Lacey

D1418939

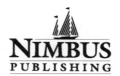

NIMBUS
PUBLISHING

Copyright © Laurie Lacey, 1993

All rights reserved. No part of this book covered by the copyrights hereon may be reproduced or used in any form or by any means—graphic, electronic or mechanical—without the prior written permission of the publisher. Any request for photocopying, recording, taping or information storage and retrieval systems of any part of this book shall be directed in writing to the Canadian Reprography Collective, 379 Adelaide Street West, Suite M1, Toronto, Ontario M5V 1S5.

Nimbus Publishing Limited
P.O. Box 9301, Station A
Halifax, Nova Scotia
B3K 5N5 (902) 455-4286

Editor: Anne Webb
Design: Kathy Kaulbach, Halifax
Illustrations: Laurie Lacey
Printed and bound in Canada

Canadian Cataloguing in Publication Data
Lacey, Laurie.
Micmac medicines
Includes bibliographical references.
ISBN 1-55109-041-4
1. Lacey, Laurie. 2. Micmac Indians—Ethnobotany. 3. Indians of North America—Maritime Provinces—Ethnobotany. 4. Materia medica, Vegetable—Maritime Provinces. I. Title.

E99.M6L32 1993   581.6'34'089973   C92-098734-6

Disclaimer
The author and publisher are not responsible for the misuse of medicinal remedies described in this book. The book is a naturalist and folklore presentation, and no attempt has been made to check the remedies medically. No reader should assume that a remedy or cure in this book has been approved and may be used without further investigation. Furthermore, caution should be used to ensure that the correct part of a plant is collected and used.

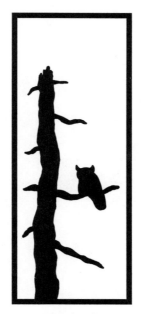

This book
is dedicated
to my cousin,
the late
Charles Richard Lacey,
with whom
I shared
many adventures.

CONTENTS

■ ■ ■ ■ ■
FOREWORD
■ ■ ■ ■ ■

I first met Laurie Lacey in 1976 when he was in the process of writing about Micmac medicines. During his visit to our home, my late husband Ben and I got to know him as a dedicated researcher of roots and herbs and how they were prepared to cure the ills of the Micmac people. Our talk was not solely about medicines at this time—a good-friend relationship was beginning to grow. We have remained good friends for sixteen years. From the time of that first contact with Laurie, my support for him and his process of learning about a part of our Micmac culture has never ceased.

I was always told by my parents that Mother Nature provides for us all whether the need is for food, shelter or clothing. It is the medicines as foods that provide good health for us regardless of our age.

The Micmac medicines originated in time immemorial, at the same time that the Micmac language was born. Different family groups in different parts of North America studied and then shared with one another ways of curing ills. A vital basic need for Micmacs was to be in good physical health in order to survive. The use of plants, roots and herbs for medicinal purposes had to be practiced in an underground fashion because of fear that the outside world and Reserve institutions would arrest this age-old basic need.

The importance of Micmac medicine in today's world helps to bind the First Nations together. That is to say that in order to keep the Nation alive it is necessary not to allow Micmac customary practices to disappear. Their use will be passed down to the present day generation, so that they in turn can do the same thing to their children and grandchildren. The realization that herbal medicines continue to be practiced by some Micmac elders gives a very strong indication that the Micmac Nation knew how to cure sicknesses and bring relief to those who suffered aches and pains. Knowledgeable elders have a role to play. I have seen the elderly sharing medicines at Pow Wows. They were helping to keep a Nation together even to the present day.

The Micmac world of today needs to learn about medicines and must be taught how they are gathered and prepared. If your interest is in Native medicines and you want to expand that interest, *Micmac Medicines: Remedies and Recollections* can put a spark into your curious mind. Then you will begin to realize why the Micmacs are a proud people.

Rose Knockwood-Morris, BSW
Gold River Micmac Reserve
December 9, 1992

■ ■ ■ ■ ■
ACKNOWLEDGEMENTS
■ ■ ■ ■ ■

I am sincerely grateful to the Micmac people who contributed their knowledge to the pages of this book. Some of these people I met only once, while others I saw on several occasions and came to call them friends. I wish to offer special thanks to Rebecca Pictou, Nancy Christoff, Sadie and William Paul, Thomas Alonzo Maloney, Joseph Louis, Rachel and Charles Marshall, Charles Labrador, Frank Jeremy, Noel McCooney, Fanny Muise, Frank and Rita Joe, Andrew Battiste, Isabelle Paul, Peter P. Denny, Noel P. Denny, Victor Jeddore, Matilda Rose, Molly MacDonald, Bill Grant, Sylvestor Jeddore, Matthew Jeddore, Millie Joe, Mike Joe and those who asked that their names not be mentioned in a publication. Thank you for allowing me into your confidence and your hearts. You have had a profound influence on my life.

I would like to thank the many people who encouraged me to write this book. I hope each of you find something of value within its pages. Peggi Thayer, with whom I have shared many adventures, gave valuable suggestions for the format of this book, and over the years has been a source of encouragement and inspiration. I must also thank Larry Willett, who played a very positive role in getting me started on the initial research, back in 1974. A thank you to Lynne Meisner for her typing services, and for sharing a glass of dandelion wine at the conclusion of her work. Finally, I would like to thank Dorothy Blythe of Nimbus for her friendly support and professional guidance.

L.L.

INTRODUCTION

This collection of reflections and remedies is both a personal journal and a folk medicine manual. It is a product of the intertwining of my experiences, the magic of nature, and a wide assortment of traditional remedies, with a focus on plant medicines. The remedies discussed are from Micmac sources, except where otherwise noted. In some cases I have had to suggest how the medicines were *probably* prepared—based on my own knowledge of plant medicine preparation—as I could not unearth specific instructions.

I have commented on the food value of certain plants such as blackberry and strawberry as dietary factors are clearly very important in the maintenance of good health. Early records indicate that in traditional Native culture, good health was generally the natural state of the people, and the result of a balanced lifestyle. Drug therapy as used in modern western medicine was not commonly required by the Micmac in the pre-contact period. Serious illnesses were treated by shamans, while minor external injuries were dressed with medicines derived from plants, trees and animal parts. Micmac knowledge of natural medicines was as effective as the knowledge of their European counterparts, and in some instances surpassed it.

The Micmac experienced frequent contact with Europeans earlier than other North American Native peoples. As early as 1500 A.D. Micmac culture was undergoing changes as a result of contact with fishing vessels and the ensuing fur trade. As the Micmac became more involved with European mariners, their seasonal activities changed and their health deteriorated. Rather than spending summers near rivers, catching and preserving fish, and gathering berries and other plant foods, the Micmac would wait near the coast for trading ships.

This change in behaviour radically altered the diet of the people, particularly during the winter months, as food stocks were small and composed mostly of hardtack and biscuits received in trade with the Europeans. According to writers such as Nicolas Denys and Marc Lescarbot, the Micmac soon became afflicted with lung, chest and intestinal disorders, and experienced a decrease in their life expectancy. As time passed, the people suffered from a broad range of diseases and ailments with which they were unfamiliar and unable to cope. To make matters worse, the Micmac were wards of the colonial government, and were forced to live in deplorable conditions.

These harsh conditions drew out the resourcefulness of the people. They gradually acquired remedies to combat ailments which were unknown a few generations earlier. It is difficult to say how this knowledge was gained. Some uses for plants were probably discovered by accident, while other remedies must have been uncovered as a result of experimentation with plants. Perhaps certain people had visions or dreams about the healing properties of particular plants and trees. Additionally, interaction between settlers and Native people would have resulted in an exchange of medicinal information. In any case, much of this knowledge was passed down through generations of Micmac people, and some of it has reached the pages of this book.

I have included illustrations of the plants discussed, but would suggest that readers use a plant identification manual as a companion to this book.[1] Those who are inspired to begin an exploration of the beautiful world of plant life should take a good manual with them and hike along a rocky shoreline to get a first-hand taste of crowberries or explore bogs and other wet areas to see the blue flag growing there. Those whose mobility is limited may need to examine the plant life closer to home. Such outdoor excursions are good for the mind, body and spirit, and will introduce you to the intrigues of natural remedies.

OLD
MEDICINE
JARS

I

When I walked into her house, the woman was weaving baskets from strips of white ash carefully piled near her chair. The aroma of sweet grass which was resting on a table nearby permeated the air.

"You're the one who wants to know about medicines," she said matter of factly.

"Yes, I'm trying to learn about plant medicines," I replied, surprised by her disarming tone.

"What you gonna do with it?" she asked. I told her that besides wanting the knowledge myself, I wished to write it down to make it available to others, and to keep it for future generations. Her response was vague and I am not certain what she thought of my idea, but she did offer me a cup of tea—the strongest cup of tea I have ever tasted.

I sipped my tea and watched her make the white ash basket. Very little was said for the next half-hour or so, although many thoughts

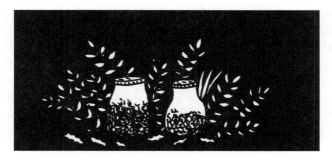

were going through my mind. I remember thinking that the woman was more serious than other people I had spoken to during my research. I was fascinated, and the more I watched her the more I respected her, and the more attentive I became to her every word.

She placed the partly finished basket on the floor and asked me to help her carry some things to her work table. We fetched some freshly gathered barks and twigs and a collection of jars containing plant materials. She opened each jar in turn, taking out a small sample and moving it between her index finger and thumb.

"You don't ever use my name when you write about the medicine," she said. "You list the medicines, that's the main thing. I don't want my name in books." I was disappointed because I wanted to give proper credit to all my "sources." But, in the end, she had her way.

She began to tell me about plants. "The sweet grass is for all the people. God gave us the grass to use in our baskets, our homes, or wherever we live. I'm a Catholic, but I still use it. Sometimes on T.V. you see the medicine man using it. But the sweet grass is for everybody, and not just for special people. My grandfather told me to hang it in the house to keep everything pure. If he was living he could tell you about it."

She handed me a jar filled with broken pieces of dried plant root and asked if I had ever seen the medicine before. She added, "It's bloodroot—you find it near wet places. I got this a couple years ago outside Truro. Some people used it for TB. But you have to be careful because its poisonous, if you use it in the wrong way." She showed me samples of plants from other containers, including prince's pine and several willows. Some of the samples were old, and must have been collected several years prior to my visit.

We went outside to find the Indian tobacco plant. We walked through the hardwood forest until we came to an old road which she said was seldom used. We followed the road to a point where it began to climb to higher ground. The trees were mostly beech, with numerous maple and birch scattered throughout, and a few conifers.

She stopped and pointed to a group of plants about eight to twelve inches tall and light green in colour. She explained that these were Indian tobacco plants, and that it is best to look for them in hardwood areas where there are clearings or on old roads. "Look for the red ground," she told me. I have not forgotten those words, and whenever I look for Indian tobacco I follow her instructions. I left her place with a better understanding of plant medicines and, more importantly, of humility; I gained a greater respect for the traditions and knowledge which some people expand into wisdom as they pass through life.

II

In Eskasoni, Cape Breton, one summer I visited a man who spoke to me about the *eptekewey*, or "hot root." This is the Micmac name for horse radish, which is rich in vitamins A and C and has a long history of usage in herbal medicine. The plant can be used as a stomach medicine, but only a small portion of the root is required as it is very strong. When I left Eskasoni my friend gave me several large horse radish plants to take home and transplant. I caught a bus to Sydney and took an Eastern Provincial Airlines flight to Halifax. I remember the startled look of the flight attendant as I entered the plane with my collection of plants. I do not think she had encountered such baggage before. But she got the plants settled comfortable and we made it back to Halifax.

After returning from Eskasoni, I went to visit a friend on the Wildcat Reserve in Queens County, Nova Scotia. He was running a summer camp for youths, and invited me to take the young people on nature walks to identify medicinal plants. During one of my visits to the camp my friend introduced me to an elderly man who knew a lot about medicines.

We entered his home in the middle of the afternoon. He offered us each a cup of Labrador tea, explaining that he always kept a pot of it on his wood stove to offer to guests. He believed the tea was an excellent tonic, and had used it himself for several years.

The elderly man was particularly fond of skunk cabbage, and talked at length about his experiences with the plant. He told us that the root was the most important part of the plant, and should be collected in early June. It would be impossible to find later in the summer because the plant rots away quickly, making the root difficult to locate. He often travelled to the Yarmouth area to collect the root as this is one of the few places in the province where the skunk cabbage grows.

Our host claimed to have cured diabetes with the root, but warned that it is strong and must be treated with respect. He remarked that years earlier a medical doctor in Bridgewater, Nova Scotia, had tried to get him to reveal his cure for diabetes, and had offered him a large sum of money, but he refused to disclose the remedy.

The root of the skunk cabbage will also cure a toothache. A piece of the root should be placed against the gum of the aching tooth. It is a rather torturous treatment, if the root has not been thoroughly dried. It causes a burning sensation akin to that of the Indian turnip which is a member of the same plant family. It is believed that if the root is applied often enough to the gum of the aching tooth, it will cause it to "drop from the mouth."

III

One year I went to Newfoundland to visit the Micmac community of Conne River, on the southwest coast of the province. I travelled there with a friend who was doing research in Newfoundland. He took me by car as far as the river which ran in front of the community. I waited there until a couple of boys noticed me and began waving to get my attention. They rowed over and brought me across the river. At the band office I explained my interest in traditional Native health practices, particularly plant medicines, and told them about my research in Nova Scotia. I found that they were interested in establishing that the Micmac in Nova Scotia and Newfoundland have similar traditions. At this time the Conne

River Micmac were trying to establish Indian status with the Canadian government.

I was given the use of a trailer to stay in and was introduced to several of the older people in the community. These people mentioned cow parsnip more frequently than most other plants. Many considered it an "all-purpose" medicine. Some stressed its importance as an internally taken medicine in the treatment of colds, influenza and tuberculosis. A few people told me that by simply wearing pieces of the root about the neck and inhaling the fumes one is able to prevent many kinds of ailments. The plant is plentiful along the Conne River, and its beautiful, large, dark green leaves make it easy to locate and identify.

The day before I left the community, I went to the river to see the salmon breaking water, which they often do during the warm summer days. I broke off several large cow parsnip leaves and pressed them between pieces of cardboard. I collected many plant samples in a similar fashion that summer, and sent part of the collection to the botanical division of the Natural Sciences Museum in Ottawa. The remainder I kept stored away in a box. I still have those plant samples. They are in good condition and preserve the warm memories of the Micmac people I encountered.

Bloodroot

The root was used to treat tuberculosis. It was steeped in water and taken internally. The leaves were used to treat rheumatism. They were probably softened and used as a poultice, or steeped in water and the liquid rubbed on the skin. Van Wart (pp. 574-75) suggests that the colour of the plant may have influenced its use. He explains that the roots were dried and worn about the neck to prevent bleeding.

Cow Parsnip

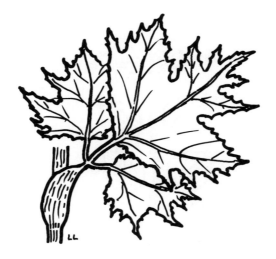

This is both a preventive medicine and a treatment for colds and influenza. It is also considered useful against tuberculosis. Wilson Wallis (p. 30) writes that when the plant is green and light in colour it is looked upon as a medicine for women; when it is dark and ripe it is considered a medicine for men. Wallis gives the Micmac term, *wabegpagosi*, for the plant, while some of the people I spoke with called it *pagosi* (pronounced "bugosi"). Most of the older people have heard about pagosi. However, it seems it is not one particular plant. I have had people tell me it is cow parsnip root, water lily root and burdock root. Perhaps pagosi simply refers to a water root, and can mean any of the above plants.

Dogwood

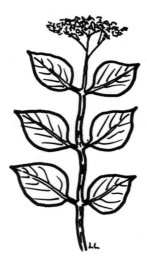

The bark of the dogwood was used
in tobacco mixtures. It was cut from
the shrub or tree, allowed to dry,
and then broken into small pieces.
This was mixed with other plants,
such as the bark and leaves of
willows, rather than smoked on its
own.

Everlasting

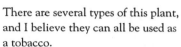

There are several types of this plant, and I believe they can all be used as a tobacco.

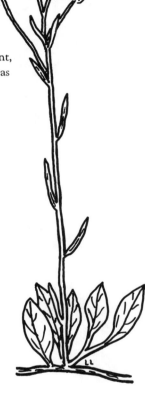

Horse Radish

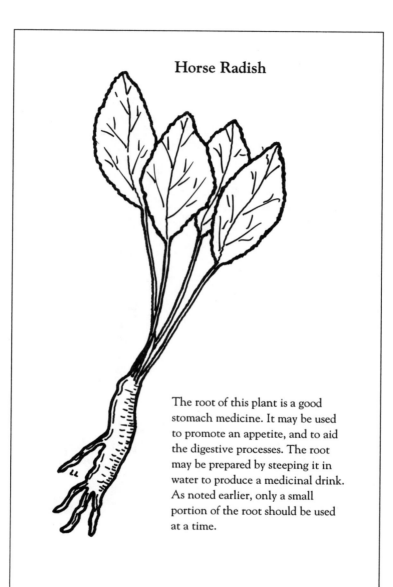

The root of this plant is a good stomach medicine. It may be used to promote an appetite, and to aid the digestive processes. The root may be prepared by steeping it in water to produce a medicinal drink. As noted earlier, only a small portion of the root should be used at a time.

Indian Tobacco

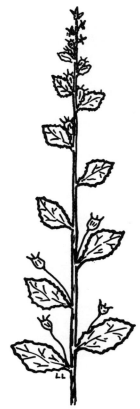

A smoking preparation is made from this plant. The smoke is known to be beneficial in treating asthma and earaches, and may have been used by the Micmac for those purposes. At one time it may also have been used for ceremonial purposes. The plant is native to North America. It contains toxic properties and must be used with much caution.

Labrador Tea

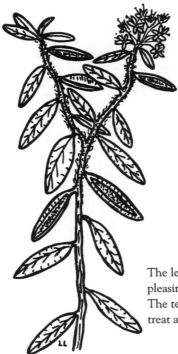

The leaves of this plant produce a
pleasing tea when steeped in water.
The tea is a tonic and was used to
treat a variety of kidney ailments.

Lady's Slipper

This plant should rarely be picked as it is an endangered plant. It was known as "moccasin flower" and as "many fine roots" by Native people.

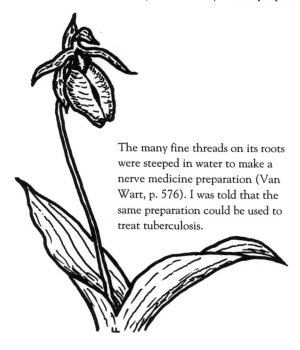

The many fine threads on its roots were steeped in water to make a nerve medicine preparation (Van Wart, p. 576). I was told that the same preparation could be used to treat tuberculosis.

Lambkill

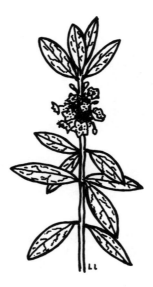

This is a poisonous plant, but it may be boiled in water and the liquid used for external purposes. It was used as a bathing solution to reduce swellings, ease the pain of rheumatism, and to treat sore legs and feet. An alternative method of treatment was rubbing freshly picked lambkill leaves on the affected areas of the body.

Prince's Pine

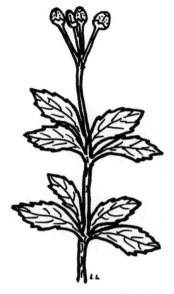

The plant was used to treat
tuberculosis. It was also considered
useful for many other ailments. I
would suggest that any well
recognized herbal guide be
consulted for a more complete
picture of this valuable medicinal
plant.

Skunk Cabbage

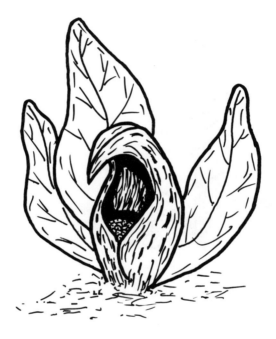

A small piece of the root of the plant was steeped in a cup of water and a teaspoon of the warm medicine was taken three times daily for a period of four to five months to treat diabetes. It was also used to cure a toothache, as explained earlier. If you wish to find the source of this plant's name, cut or bruise some of its leaves. An obnoxious odour much like that given off by a skunk will be released.

Sweet Grass

This plant has great ceremonial and spiritual value in Native culture. It is used for purification purposes.

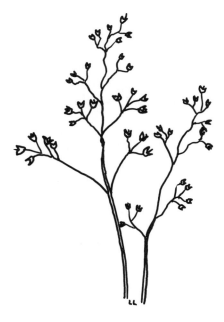

Pussy Willow

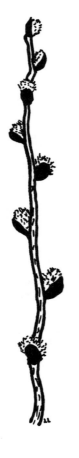

For external use, the bark peelings should be boiled to a thick molasses-like state. It can be used in poultice form to treat bruises, lame areas of the body and skin cancer. For internal use, the peelings should be steeped as a tea and taken to treat colds and kidney ailments. The bark of certain willows, such as the red willow, was dried and used in tobacco mixtures.

REMEDIES
FROM
SWAMPS AND BOGS

Swamps and bogs are places we rarely visit. As children we are told not to visit those places mostly because we will return with mud stained trousers, water-logged socks, and sneakers which give off a variety of obnoxious swampy odours. But I was a determined child and often would visit a special swamp which was replete with alder bushes of many shapes and sizes.

The swamp was located by a steep out-cropping of rock. It was a ten minute walk from my home, along an old dirt mining road. When I first discovered it, I found a large metal container neatly tucked away against the base of the rock. I used it for drumming. I was in love with the Australian aborigines, and would perform drumming songs which sounded throughout the area.

I never discovered why the drum was placed there. My parents did not seem to know. Then again, perhaps they were not telling me everything. As I later realized, the container may have been used to

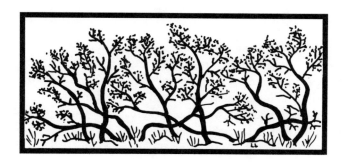

Remedies from Swamps and Bogs

store home-made brew or moonshine. When I visited that swamp recently the metal drum was still there, exactly as it was during my childhood.

My swamp was alive with moss, many varieties of plants, ferns, and alders which formed a jungle-like network of branches across the breadth of the area. A favourite game was trying to cross the swamp without getting wet feet. My friend and I would attempt to walk on the alder branches, moving carefully from branch to branch until we could go no further. We would then retreat and try again from another location.

It was easy moving along those branches which grew low across the surface of the swamp. We had greater difficulty with the ones which required bending. We bent them over with our hands and stepped on them, applying pressure with out feet while clutching higher branches with our hands for balance and support. You can imagine the spring-like force beneath our feet. I often found myself stretched to the limit, and often ended up with a wet rear-end.

Later in life I came to realize the many gifts alder has to offer, medicinal and otherwise. Beautiful rustic furniture can be made from peeled alder branches, and a rich orange-red dye can be made from the inner bark. Alder was used by the Micmac for medicinal purposes, and is found in the folk medicine traditions of many peoples. In the last century, rural people of the Alps are said to have cured cases of rheumatism by covering their patients with bags of heated alder leaves. The Micmac at Conne River used the leaves in the same manner. I discuss this further in the plant notes section below.

There is a swamp near my cabin which I visit in the winter when its surface is frozen and it is possible to explore the full extent of its landscape. It is a special place where many kinds of medicines can be found if you look closely, and are not distracted by little things such as rabbit tracks which are found there. I visit when the weather is cold and the sun is bright, near mid-morning, when the eastern light causes the frost to sparkle. There is often a calm stillness about a swamp in the winter, especially if it is sheltered from the north wind. But the stillness is fragile and easily broken by the utterance of a crow or raven, or some other bird. Sound travels rapidly in the clear, crisp winter air. Swamp grasses are brittle, snapping between boot and ice. If you listen to the sound you will hear the echo of your footsteps in the forest ahead of you.

Alder

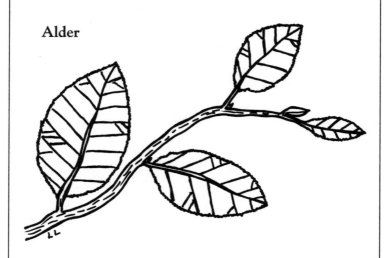

The Micmac steeped the bark from alders in water and used the tea to treat stomach cramps, kidney ailments, fever and neuralgic pain. It was also a common Micmac remedy for diphtheria. The bark and leaves were used together in poultice form as a treatment for festering wounds.

In Conne River, a man told me alder was good for treating lameness in the body. He said that when he was young he was very lame. At one time it became so debilitating that he crawled to his dory and rowed to see a doctor in the nearby community of St. Albans. The doctor told him there was no cure for the condition. Later, he met someone who offered to help him overcome his crippling condition. The individual collected a large bag of alder leaves and spent the following night treating the problem. The leaves were placed over the affected areas of the body, and were replaced with a fresh covering whenever they became "too hot." This cured the lameness.

Blue Flag

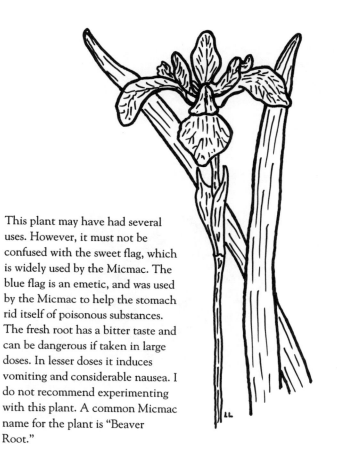

This plant may have had several uses. However, it must not be confused with the sweet flag, which is widely used by the Micmac. The blue flag is an emetic, and was used by the Micmac to help the stomach rid itself of poisonous substances. The fresh root has a bitter taste and can be dangerous if taken in large doses. In lesser doses it induces vomiting and considerable nausea. I do not recommend experimenting with this plant. A common Micmac name for the plant is "Beaver Root."

Cranberry

The berries, stewed, make an excellent sauce. They can be steeped in water to make a general potable tonic.

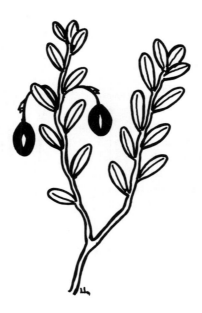

Cranberry
(Highbush)

This bush was sometimes called the
"flat seed berry" plant. The berries
were used to make a beverage. Also,
the plant was used to treat swollen
glands (Van Wart, p. 576).

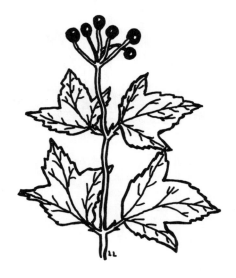

Pitcher Plant

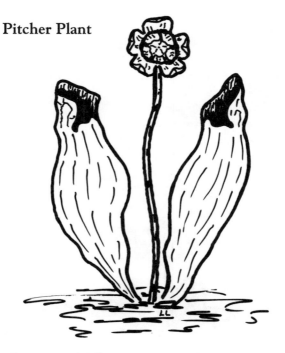

When I was a child I was fascinated by the pitcher plant. I would examine the cup-like parts of the plant, paying particular attention to the kinds of insects trapped therein, and wondering if there was something special about the water within those cups. The water was a magic elixir, but I was always afraid to taste it. The Micmac call the plant "Indian Cut Root." It was used to treat tuberculosis during the early part of this century. The root is believed to be effective in treating kidney ailments. It was also used to relieve indigestion. The root should be steeped in water and the medicine taken in small doses.

Sweet Flag

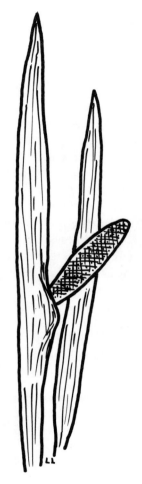

This plant has a long history of usage in both Native and non-Native folk medicine traditions. The Micmac considered it a preventive medicine. They would place the root in water and steam it in the home to prevent illness. It was also carried on the person to prevent disease. I know a man who sewed it into his shirt collar for this purpose. The root was also chewed to relieve indigestion and stomach cramps. Sometimes it was powdered and mixed with warm water and taken in this fashion. The medicine was given to infants to ease stomach pain, cramps and belching. Many years ago it may have been used to treat cholera. Common Micmac terms for the plant are "Flagroot" and "Muskrat Food."

A MEDICINE WALK
IN THE
BARRENS

There is a mood or a special atmosphere in the barrens. It is especially strong near large boulders, exposed rock ledges and places where wind-swept pines cling to rocks, gaining sustenance from whatever soil is available. This feeling will not escape you, and you will want to return to the barrens often. Some places are like that. They leave us with haunting impressions for the rest of our lives.

The barrens, located in the vicinity of Bridgewater, Nova Scotia, is named for its rocky terrain. The ledges of gold-bearing bedrock run north to south throughout the area. In some places the boulders, split open by the action of natural forces, lie like guardians over the landscape.

A fire devastated the barrens in 1955. I was only six years old, so I can only imagine how desolate it must have looked afterwards. A pillar of black smoke was clearly visible to the north, and I remember watching my parents and neighbours loading our belongings on a truck, just in case we had to evacuate our home.

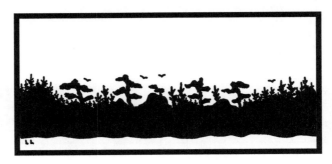

Evidence of the fire remains, although it is less obvious with each passing year. If you hike in that country, you will find the occasional blackened old stump. If you examine the ground carefully you will find bits of old charcoal. Those are memories which the landscape will not give up.

My father was one of the people who fought the fire. He often mentions the frightening experience of being trapped by the flames. He and a buddy were forced to stand up to their waists in water in a small cove to escape the fire while windswept flames closed in around them, sending its deadly heat, burning cinders and choking smoke down upon them.

There are tall pines in the barrens. They are not particularly large, but are very straight. The pines are plentiful near the lakes, and contrast sharply with the other trees there, some of which are peculiar shapes. Certain trees shape themselves to the contour of the land and are especially affected by the strong winds which sweep over the barrens from the west or northwest. In the past moose would roam amongst those trees and drink from Leipsigaek Lake. But now the moose are only visible at dusk when their ghosts emerge with the last waves of light which pass over the barren rocks.

The Leipsigaek Gold Fields are in the barrens. When the largest of the mines was in operation, the area was teeming with prospectors, miners and shop keepers and their families. People from many parts of North America found their way there to search for gold or to work in the mines.

There are different explanations for how gold was first discovered in the barrens. I was told that Sarah Weagle went for her cows one evening and got lost. While trying to find her way, she came to several large white boulders which must have been quartz. The incident was talked about until it reached the ears of Lewis and John Labrador. They came prospecting and discovered a main gold bearing lead. Because the men were Micmac it became known as the Micmac lead, and the mine as the Micmac Gold Mine. Eventually, other mines worked the same lead.

My father was a prospector and gold miner, as was my grandfather before him. They spent many of their working years in the gold fields. My grandfather is supposed to have had the ability to find gold where other people could not—it was a family secret, passed down through the generations.

I have hiked much of the barren country. When I went there with my father he pointed out where many of the old mines are located. We walked to the location of a gold bearing lead, which he found near Leipsigaek Lake. The lead has never been worked. It dips into the ground and runs beneath the bedrock.

My father is now too old to walk in the barrens, but I have gathered some of his stories, and the stories of other people who lived there. There are other stories in the barrens which remain untold, and are waiting to be collected. This is why I often go there. I am convinced that the "special mood" of the place will unlock these stories, which could fill several journals.

There are many old roads in the barrens, several of which lead to abandoned mines or to lakes in the area. There is one particular road on the way to Leipsigaek Lake which runs past a place where the mullein plant grows. The plant has been growing there for several years now near a section which was built from crushed mining rock. Here poison ivy also grows on both sides of the road. It seems to encroach more onto the road with each passing year. Nearby there is a swamp with alder bushes throughout, and close to the road is a grassy spot and an old apple tree. There must have been a building in that location at some time in the past.

I found the mullein plant on the shoulder of the road, rooted in the crushed mining rock. Its velvet-like woolly leaves are easy to recognize as they form a rosette during the initial year of growth. In the second year, a single flower stalk grows from the centre of this rosette. The plant appears to thrive in places where it is exposed to a lot of heat and sun.

The mullein is scattered in the barrens, and I know of only a few places where it is growing. I saw it near the old Micmac mine in a sandy field. The field is composed of crushed rock which has gone through the milling process. This turns the rock into fine sand. The other place I found the plant was near the Minamkeak Lake dam. This was the largest mullein I have ever seen. It must have been seven feet tall.

Beyond where the mullein plant grows, there is a fork in the road. Leipsigaek Lake lies half a mile along the right fork. The shoreline is very rocky, and at certain places veins of quartz run through the rock. I go there every autumn to pick a supply of cranberries for the Christmas dinner. They are rich in vitamin C and are excellent for jam and jelly. At Leipsigaek the berries are plentiful and there are places where they form a beautiful red carpet over and around rocks, grasses and other plants.

The boneset plant is also scattered along the shore of Leipsigaek Lake and is a neighbour of the cranberry. It is easy to identify and should be collected in late summer or early autumn.

I went to Leipsigaek last September to gather boneset plants. While collecting them I noticed the fresh tracks of a doe deer in the soft mud. I followed the tracks for quite a distance along the edge of the lake until they turned inland. At that point I gave up tracking the doe and decided to climb a bluff which afforded a good view of the lake.

I sat to the left of a witch hazel tree and looked over the cove to the other shore. It was a clear autumn day. I saw a single leaf fall from a beech tree near the distant shoreline. It seemed to flutter in slow motion.

There are several birch trees on the bluff. Their leaves spoke with "clicking" voices as a breeze came up from the southwest. The trees stirred by the far shore. While walking home from the lake I kicked my boots through the deep layers of dry leaves. In the evening I found a single beech leaf on my cabin floor.

Bearberry

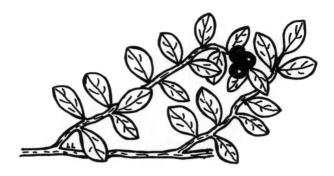

The leaves and/or berries steeped in water make an excellent general potable tonic which has an antiseptic effect on the urinary passages. Bearberry is sometimes referred to as kinnikinnick in plant manuals. However, others claim that kinnikinnick is a compound mixture, and that the bearberry leaf is one of its ingredients.

Boneset

This plant is easy to recognize because the sessile and bases of the two opposite leaves are united. I am referring to *Eupatorium perfoliatum*.

The *trifolium* Fassett type has three leaves at a node rather than the usual two. The boneset is used for a variety of purposes. In folk medicine it is taken as a general tonic and for relief from arthritic pain. A Micmac woman told me it may be used to treat stomach ulcers. I have used it to treat a cold, and have noticed if taken at bed time it is very relaxing and promotes a sound sleep.

Juniper
(Common)

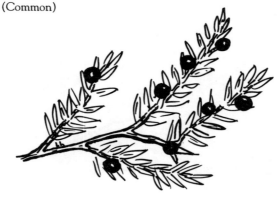

This plant is very common in the Maritime provinces. The Micmac used juniper for many purposes. The gum was used to heal cuts, sores, burns and sprains, and to treat colds and influenza. The tips of juniper branches were steeped in water to make a beverage. The inner bark and juice were used to treat stomach ulcers. The former would be steeped in water and taken as a tea. Juniper roots were referred to as "rheumatism roots," and were considered very effective for treating the problem. The roots were probably steeped in water and the liquid rubbed on the rheumatic area, or mixed into a salve for this purpose. The plant was also used to treat kidney ailments and as a urinary tract medicine.

A Micmac woman at Shubenacadie said that juniper tea was a good all-purpose tonic. She said the entire plant should be steeped in water and that it is best to collect the plant in the autumn, near apple picking season. Steep it until the water turns colour.

Mullein
(Common)

This plant was introduced from Europe. It has a long history of use in herbal medicine. Maud Grieve, in her *A Modern Herbal* (p. 564), writes that before the introduction of cotton, the "down" on the leaves and stem was used to make lamp wicks. There is an old folk belief, according to Grieve, that witches used lamps and candles with wicks of this kind during their incantations.

The Micmac used the leaves of the mullein to treat asthma. They were smoked for this purpose, or steeped in water, and the fumes inhaled. I do not recommend drinking tea made from mullein leaves. There are fine hairs on the leaves, and if those get in the tea they may cause throat irritation.

Pine
(White)

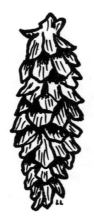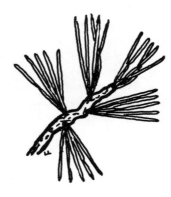

The bark, needles and twigs were steeped in water and the tea drunk as a remedy for colds. The same preparation was probably used to treat kidney problems. Other types of pines may have been used for similar purposes. Wilson Wallis (p. 26) writes that the sap and juice of the pine bark mixed with warm water was taken to treat hemorrhaging. Wallis does not refer to any particular type of pine and, in fact, may be referring to the hackmatack tree which has astringent properties and is a member of the pine family.

Poplar

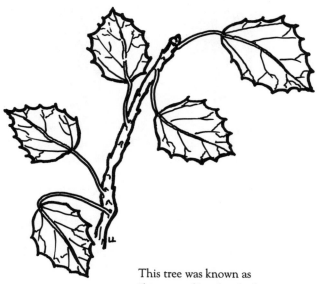

This tree was known as "bitterwood" and its bark was steeped in water, as a medicine for colds and influenza. Poplar bark was also used to treat worms in animals and humans. The bark was baked until brown, scraped into a powder, and probably used as a tea. When treating animals, the powder may have been mixed with food.

Spruce

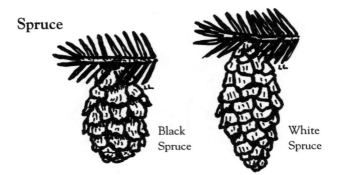

Black Spruce

White Spruce

When my father worked in the woods cutting pulpwood he used to make tea from spruce twigs. The Micmac may have used spruce to treat scurvy. The bark of the black spruce was used to make a tonic. A friend in Eskasoni told me that her husband used to suffer a great deal with laryngitis. She said that the medical specialist was unable to help him. Someone told him to chew the inner bark of the spruce tree. He did this on a regular basis. He even carried pieces of the bark to work with him in his lunch box. After a number of weeks it cured the laryngitis. The bark was probably from the black spruce tree

An elderly man at Millbrook told me that the inner bark of the spruce is a good weight reducing tonic. When I visited him we went into the woods and collected an arm load of the bark for this purpose. He said that his wife was going to use it to reduce her weight. The inner bark is steeped in water and several cups of the brew drunk daily.

The white spruce (cat spruce) was used to treat infections of various kinds. The bark was steeped in water or chewed. At one time it was used to treat tuberculosis. I imagine the inner bark and/or twigs were used.

WILD BLACKBERRY
AND OTHER
MEDICINAL PLANTS

When I began my research on the uses of plants as medicines, my knowledge of plant life was limited. I was able to identify a few common plants, but found it difficult to follow many of the things the Native people were saying about plants. I knew that if I was to be successful in my project, I would have to gain a deeper understanding of local plant life.

During the summer of 1974, my brother and I spent much of our time in the field with a manual, learning to identify plants. Whenever we found a particularly interesting plant we would locate it in the manual and study its characteristics. Often we would spend hours investigating a few plants. Our efforts proved worthwhile, and I would recommend this approach to anyone wanting to gain a greater appreciation of local flora.

As I advanced in my study, I became acutely aware of plant communities. I examined the nature of the soils in which plants

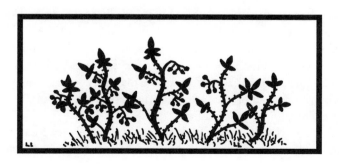

Wild Blackberry and Other Medicinal Plants

grow and made mental notes about the types of plants I found growing together. I found that certain plants always grow near particular kinds of trees. These types of observations are valuable to the plant naturalist.

Near my cabin is a section of forest I call the "medicine woods." This is where I go to collect many of my favourite medicinal plants. Wild blackberries grow here. They appeared several years ago when part of the forest was logged. The brambles grew up through the piles of brush which were left in the cut area. They were plentiful, as was their close relative, the raspberry, as both plants like to grow in this sort of environment.

Today the blackberries are not so plentiful, having been replaced by young hardwood growth. However, scattered clumps remain, as does the occasional raspberry stalk. Wild blackberries have approximately the same food value as domestic fruits such as apples, oranges and peaches, per equal serving. They also compare very well to other fruits in terms of protein and carbohydrates. Blackberries are rich in calcium, potassium and vitamins A and C. This is also true for wild raspberries; most wild berries compare favourably with domestic fruits in terms of food value, vitamins and minerals.

There are few berries as delicious as the wild strawberry. I have yet to taste a domestic strawberry that can match the wild varieties. The wild berry is high in food value and is one of the easiest plants to collect for herbal purposes. I have only to step outside my cabin door to collect the plants.

Blueberries are also plentiful where I live. There are several kinds of blueberries, and it is often difficult to distinguish between them. Furthermore, the different varieties commonly cross-pollinate and hybrids occur. This is of no great concern to me as I am not a professional botanist. Yet, I do consider myself a connoisseur of fine blueberries, and admit that I am slightly biased in favour of the taste of the large, juicy, dark variety.

However, I will usually pick and eat any blueberry I can find, except for one type: the half dry bead-like berries which from a distance look like a woven blue carpet. They are small and seem to dry as soon as they ripen. I am sure they are berries which have fallen victim to certain climatic conditions. In any case, they are a terrible disappointment to someone like myself, who enjoys a long list of blueberry delights, ranging from blueberry pie to fine flavoured blueberry wine.

The blueberry has a high food value and contains a number of vitamins and minerals, including iron. In Lunenburg County, Nova Scotia, a favourite berry dish is "Blueberry Grunt." This is made from layers of blueberries and biscuit dough, with sugar sprinkled on each layer and moistened with water. It is then cooked over the stove for approximately twenty minutes, without removing the cover from the pot. If you remove the cover while cooking, the dough will get soggy or heavy. This is a delicious way to eat blueberries and is a recipe any connoisseur will appreciate.

Blackberry

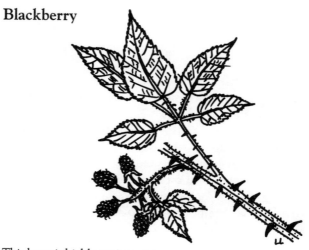

This berry is highly astringent, which makes it useful in treating diarrhoea. The entire plant may be used for this purpose, although the root has the highest astringency. The "runners" make a good stomach medicine. I was told that they should be broken up and steeped in water for this purpose. The thorns must be carefully removed from the runners before preparing the medicine. The tea is soothing to the stomach. The leaves and berries steeped in water also make a multipurpose tonic which can be used to heal cankers or sores of the mouth or throat.

Blueberry

The leaves and/or root of this plant can be used to treat rheumatism. They may be boiled in water and the liquid rubbed on the painful area of the body. The berries themselves act as a good general tonic.

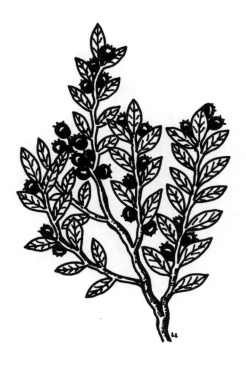

Raspberry

The same applies as for the
blackberry.

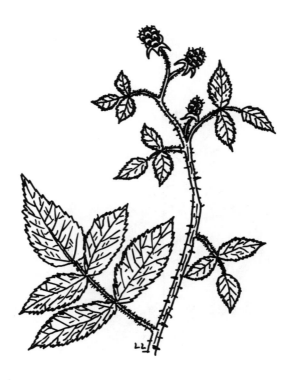

Strawberry

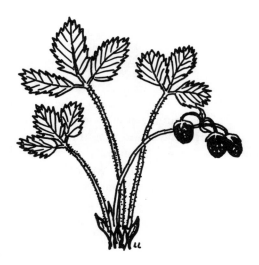

I have used strawberry leaves to treat stomach cramps. The leaves may be chewed or steeped in water to produce a medicinal tea. A Micmac woman in Shubenacadie remarked that the entire strawberry plant when steeped in water is a good general tonic. The leaves, roots and berries steeped in water make a blood purifying medicine and act as a blood building agent. Also, the plant can be used to treat dysentery and weakness of the intestines, as well as infections of the urinary organs. There are other uses for the strawberry plant. For example, a strong tea used as a gargle will strengthen the gums. (See the *Micmac News*, September 1974, p. 20 for additional uses.)

MEDICINAL BARKS
AND
WINTER BEECH

I

We walked rapidly over the frozen ground towards a stand of young beech trees. She was a Micmac woman in her mid fifties, and had spent most of a fine January afternoon talking to me about her childhood in Shubenacadie, and about her parents.

"My mother was always collecting barks and other things, when people were sick. It didn't seem to matter what time of year it was, she could always find medicines. I remember going out with her one winter when my brother had a bad fever, and finding some barks," she told me as we neared the beech trees.

"My mother usually only gathered barks when she had a use for them.[2] She had many beliefs about medicines. I suppose nowadays people would call her superstitious," the women remarked, laughing. "She believed that if you collected medicines when you didn't need them, you were inviting sickness into your life. I was only a young girl when she showed me how to take medicine bark from a tree."

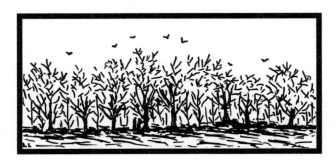

"She used to pray before she did anything else. My mother had strong faith. Then she collected the medicines. She would always use bark from the part of the tree on which the sun was shining, and gathered it in the morning or early afternoon if she could. Mother always said to get the bark from the east or south sides of the tree, because it was the best for medicine."

The woman took her knife and peeled a strip of bark from a young beech, to illustrate how to take bark from a tree. She emphasized that it should be cut, peeled or scraped in a motion away from the body and towards the roots. "This shows that the illness is leaving the body of the sick person," she explained. The healing process began with the gathering and preparation of the medicines.

As I watched her gather the beech bark, my mind flashed back to an incident my father told me about. It happened many years ago when he was sick with tuberculosis. A Micmac woman who lived near the town of Bridgewater, Nova Scotia, told him to collect "winter beech" leaves for his illness. She said the winter beech was the beech tree which retained its dried leaves over the winter months. I do not know how much of the medicine my father used, but he always spoke highly of her advice.

II

Several years ago I did a painting of hardwoods in winter which I remember fondly today. What I recall most about the painting is the way the sunlight moves from left to right across the canvas, and through the hardwood forest. I captured the warmth of March in that painting. When I did it, perhaps I was thinking of those days in late winter when you can relax in a sheltered place, away from the wind and watch the snow melt at your feet.

There is a yellow birch in the lower right corner of the painting. I placed it there to indicate the scarcity of the species in southwestern Nova Scotia. Its decline is probably the result of indiscriminate cutting practices and disease. The yellow birch has many medicinal properties; its bark was used in many Native cultures across North America.

III

When I was a young boy I fished for white perch in Minamkeak Lake. I had several favourite fishing spots, and most spring evenings I would quickly finish my school work, grab my fishing gear and walk to one of those locations. I paid particular attention during the last hour before sunset because it was the best time for catching perch.

There is a large oak tree by the shore of the lake near a spot where I used to fish. The tree is very old. When I look at it standing tall and dignified, I am reminded that the oak was considered sacred by some ancient peoples. The Druids, for example, revered the oak, and it also found a place in Christian traditions.

The medicinal value of oaks has long been recognized. It appears in old medical texts. The bark is very astringent and was used in parts of Western Europe to treat hemorrhaging. The older herbalists used the thin skin which covers the acorn to treat the spitting of blood, and acorn powder was taken in wine as a diuretic (see Grieve, p. 596). The Native people of North America used oak acorns as food. They are rich in carbohydrates and fat, and can be made into flour by grinding the dried kernels.

IV

Cedar trees are rare in Nova Scotia, but are more common in New Brunswick. The small glands of the cedar contain turpentine; this substance is responsible for its beautiful fragrance. Maud Grieve writes that *thuja*, the latin term for cedar, means "to fumigate" and comes from the Greek word *thuo*, meaning "to sacrifice" (p. 176). Apparently the fragrant wood was burned during sacrifices by ancient peoples of the Mediterranean region. The purifying nature of cedar is likely to be evident to anyone who uses it.

Other trees of importance, medicinally, include balsam fir and hackmatack. Last February I visited a bog in my medicine woods and noticed the many hackmatack growing there. Some of the trees are small but have the appearance of being old. Roland and Smith (p. 43) write that hackmatack are common in bogs, and are "one of the few tree-forms in peat bogs, where stunted individuals a few feet high may be almost 100 years old."

Beech

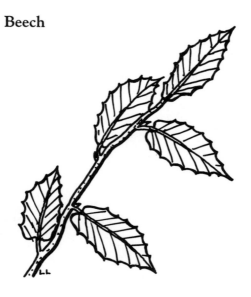

Some beech retain their dried leaves throughout the winter
months. Those leaves were steeped in water to produce a
medicinal tea which was taken to treat tuberculosis and other
chest complaints. Honey may be added to the tea to enhance
the flavour. The bark and leaves of beech have antiseptic
qualities. They can be steeped in water and taken internally as
a general tonic. The leaves are soothing to the nerves and
stomach, and help to increase one's appetite. Apparently, the
beech contains substances which are good for the liver,
kidneys and bladder, and is useful in treating intestinal
infections (see the *Micmac News*, September 1974, p.20).

Birch
(Yellow)

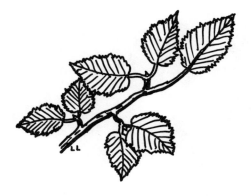

The Micmac used the bark of the yellow birch to treat rheumatism. It was steeped in water and the liquid rubbed on the rheumatic parts of the body. The inner bark of the tree was used to relieve indigestion and stomach cramps. The bark was chewed or steeped and taken as a tea. The inner bark is supposed to be nourishing and can be chewed when one is out in the woods and in need of extra energy.

This tree also provides a remedy for diarrhoea. An old man in Millbrook, Nova Scotia, told me about the remedy in the following way: "In my younger years I worked in the woods with my grandfather. One time I got the bowels running something awful! I had to run every five minutes. My grandfather helped me to find the bark of yellow birch. It cured my cramps and diarrhoea."

Cedar

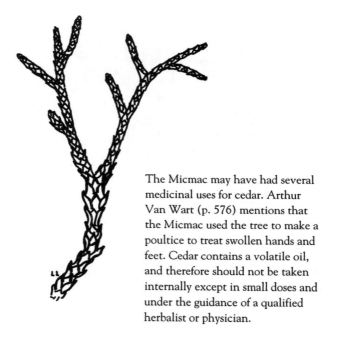

The Micmac may have had several medicinal uses for cedar. Arthur Van Wart (p. 576) mentions that the Micmac used the tree to make a poultice to treat swollen hands and feet. Cedar contains a volatile oil, and therefore should not be taken internally except in small doses and under the guidance of a qualified herbalist or physician.

Cherry

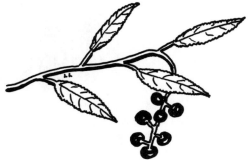

The cherry is a member of the rose family (*Rosaceae*). Parts of cherry trees are among the most frequently used and written about folk medicines in North America. The black cherry is used by the Micmac as a remedy for coughs and colds. The bark is steeped in water or simply chewed (probably the inner bark). The berries of the black cherry were steeped to make a bitter tonic. When I visited the Micmac community of Conne River, wild black cherry medicines were perhaps the most commonly cited remedies. Young and old people alike knew how to prepare the medicines.

A man in Millbrook told me that the inner bark of the red cherry may have been used to prevent high blood pressure. The bark was steeped in water and taken as a tea. The Micmac may have used the red cherry tree to treat coughs and colds, but I have no field notes to confirm this.

Chokecherry, or "bitterberry wood," was used to treat diarrhoea. The bark was steeped in water and taken as a tea (probably the inner bark). It may also have been used as a cough medicine.

Fir
(Balsam)

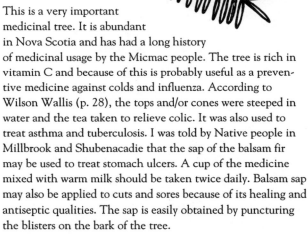

This is a very important
medicinal tree. It is abundant
in Nova Scotia and has had a long history
of medicinal usage by the Micmac people. The tree is rich in
vitamin C and because of this is probably useful as a preventive medicine against colds and influenza. According to
Wilson Wallis (p. 28), the tops and/or cones were steeped in
water and the tea taken to relieve colic. It was also used to
treat asthma and tuberculosis. I was told by Native people in
Millbrook and Shubenacadie that the sap of the balsam fir
may be used to treat stomach ulcers. A cup of the medicine
mixed with warm milk should be taken twice daily. Balsam sap
may also be applied to cuts and sores because of its healing and
antiseptic qualities. The sap is easily obtained by puncturing
the blisters on the bark of the tree.

In Conne River an elderly man told me that around the
time of the First World War there was an outbreak of
influenza, or the "grip," which caused the death of many
people in Newfoundland. He said that during the epidemic he
awoke one morning to find that he was unable to eat or speak.
Now, it happened that his father had been tanning hides in a
large wooden tub, and had used the bark and roots of the
balsam fir for this purpose. It produces a red dye. He said that
he drank a cupful of the solution, and that it cleared his throat
and chest of congestion. He finished his story by saying that
since that day he has had much respect for the medicinal
qualities of the balsam fir tree.

Hackmatack

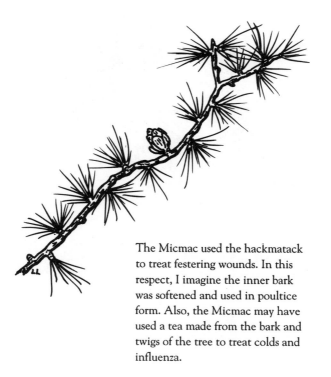

The Micmac used the hackmatack to treat festering wounds. In this respect, I imagine the inner bark was softened and used in poultice form. Also, the Micmac may have used a tea made from the bark and twigs of the tree to treat colds and influenza.

Hemlock

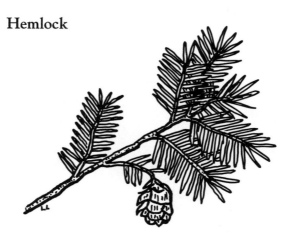

The bark of this tree was used to treat colds. It was steeped in water and the medicine taken as a tea. The hemlock tree contains a volatile oil and must be used with caution.

Oak

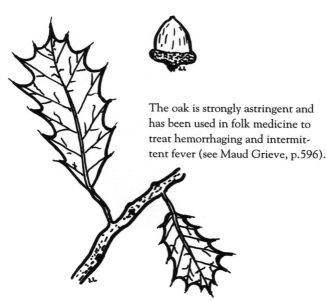

The oak is strongly astringent and has been used in folk medicine to treat hemorrhaging and intermittent fever (see Maud Grieve, p.596).

It has many other uses as well. I have read that the Micmac used the bark to treat bleeding piles. It is said that they ate the acorns of the white oak to promote thirst, as drinking a lot of water was considered beneficial to one's health (Van Wart, pp. 574-75).

Sumach
(Staghorn)

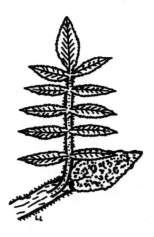

This tree was used in folk medicine to treat coughs and sore throats. The tree is closely related to poison ivy. There are hundreds of species of sumach in the world. The non-poisonous kinds of sumach can be distinguished from the poisonous types as the fruit of the former is covered with acid, crimson hairs, while their panicles are compound, dense and terminal. The poisonous varieties have smooth fruit and axillary panicles (Grieve, p.779). The Micmac used the sumach to treat earaches. Parts of the tree would be steeped in water, and the cooled liquid applied in the ear.

RECOLLECTIONS FROM THE MEDICINE WOODS

Autumn,
Leaves fall from hardwoods,
Rust and orange-red,
Near my cabin.
Stalks of
Wild sarsaparilla
Vanish from the medicine woods,
Touched by frost on the new moon.

Autumn,
I feel the chill,
I smell the breath,
I see the cool Prussian blue water
of Minamkeak Lake.
I search favourite places
For wild sarsaparilla,
Fearing it has returned
To dust in the earth.

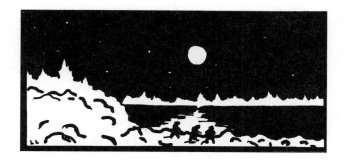

Recollections from the Medicine Woods

Autumn,
I hear it in wind through spruce trees,
Branches brush my jacket,
Needles touch my cheek.
I search my mind,
I call for wild sarsaparilla,
A soft prayer,
Deep within Self.

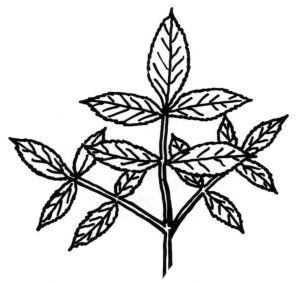

Autumn,
Vivid colours on a hillside,
Leaves strewn on granite rocks,
I see you wild sarsaparilla.
Stalks, a gold ochre,
Dance in evening wind,
One last greeting
Before winter.

II
The medicine woods,
Conifer covered,
Carpeted in moss
And beds of golden thread.
Memories of the 1950s,
Of my father collecting the long threads,
A fascinated six year old
Touched by the mystery of plants.

Old woman
Finger touching west wind,
Pointing to golden thread,
Speaking words in my ear.
Grey haired woman,
You teach this one thing,
Hands reach out for golden thread,
Sinking deep into the earth.

Grandmother,
With the soft eyes,
Laughing at granddaughter,
Sharing tea with me.
Golden thread,
Resting on window sill,
Witness to
A medicine story.

Recollections from the Medicine Woods

III

I walk the shore
Of Leipsigaek,
I walk at dusk,
I search for witch hazel.
Owl on spruce tree,
Observes movement,
I see it briefly,
It flies away.

Leipsigaek,
West wind sends waves
Splashing on shore,
I see witch hazel.
As dusk approaches
I rest on sphagnum moss,
I lie back
Against the sky.

Moon over tree line
At Leipsigaek,
Owl with large wing span
Hidden from view.
I walk the shore,
I leave that place,
Rocks under feet make clicking sounds,
Grandmothers walk in front of me.

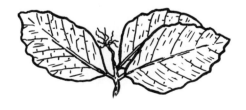

Gold Thread

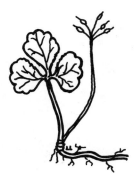

This is a popular herbal medicine in many parts of the world. In China it is used as a tonic and to stimulate the appetite. The latter is very appropriate as the plant is one of the best "bitters" to be found in the forest. The Micmac used it for this purpose, and to treat sore or chapped lips and mouth ulcers. Other uses for the plant included treating diarrhoea and diabetes. However, I know of only one instance where the plant was used for diabetes.

One individual used gold thread to treat his stomach cancer. He had terminal cancer and told me, "I took sick and had to go to the hospital. After a while the doctors let me go home. I went out in the wilds around this time [January] and I dug into the ground and found some golden threads. I steeped them in a quart of water. I took a teaspoonful every day for a month. My stomach has been good ever since. The medicine can be stored in the fridge in a container."

Wild Sarsaparilla

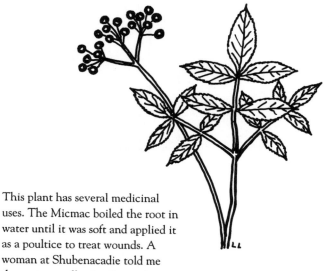

This plant has several medicinal uses. The Micmac boiled the root in water until it was soft and applied it as a poultice to treat wounds. A woman at Shubenacadie told me the root was effective in treating colds and influenza. She explained it should be dried, powdered, and steeped in water as a herbal tea. The root has a sweet spicy taste and a pleasant smell, and I suspect a certain amount of food value. This is also true for the berries, although they are not very palatable.

Witch Hazel

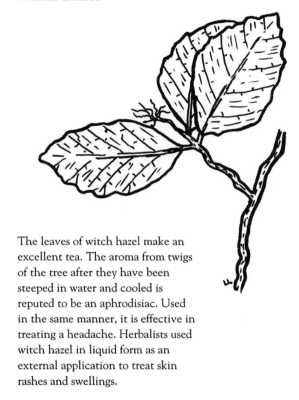

The leaves of witch hazel make an excellent tea. The aroma from twigs of the tree after they have been steeped in water and cooled is reputed to be an aphrodisiac. Used in the same manner, it is effective in treating a headache. Herbalists used witch hazel in liquid form as an external application to treat skin rashes and swellings.

SEGABUN, THE INDIAN TURNIP

I

The *segabun*, or Indian turnip, is the Micmac term for the Jack-in-the-pulpit plant. It is beautiful when fully grown, reaching approximately three feet in height, with its spike enclosed in a canopied hood. This last characteristic gives the appearance of a preacher standing in a pulpit, hence the name of the plant.

I have seen the segabun in the Hants County area—it is probably more plentiful there than in other parts of Nova Scotia. It does not grow in my medicine woods, and would seem to be totally absent from southern Nova Scotia.

I first learned about segabun while I was taking a course in ethnohistory, where I met Larry, a tall robust forest ranger. When he found out about my interest in medicinal plants, he told me about the Indian turnip. He said it was a medicinal plant and that we could find it growing near his home in Enfield. He also mentioned that a Native friend still used segabun as medicine. I visited Larry and his family in Enfield on a number of occasions.

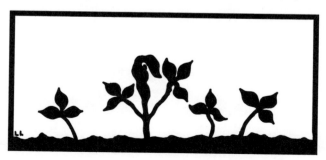

I will always remember when Larry first showed me the segabun growing in a low, swampy area near his home, and the evening he introduced me to his friend and spoke to him about my interest in Native uses of plants. Alonzo considered for a moment, said a few words in Micmac to a neighbour who was visiting that evening, and then proceeded to tell me about the medicinal uses for gold thread.

I met Alonzo on several occasions, and always wrote notes about my visits. Getting to know Alonzo was quite eventful. One evening Larry and I arrived at Alonzo's place shortly after dark. The lights were off in the cabin. We found a note nailed to the door which read, "Out in woods, back soon." I felt distraught. Larry explained that when Alonzo left a note it could mean that he would be away for the evening, or for the week! But Alonzo's home was always open to visitors so I made myself at home. Larry returned to Enfield.

Later that evening, I was relaxing with a book when a dog began barking. I was surprised as I did not know Alonzo had a dog. The barking grew more desperate and I got the impression the dog was doing its best to break down the door. I braced it with a chair. Eventually the dog quit barking. I crawled into my sleeping bag and the wind carried me off to sleep.

In the morning I washed in the brook which flowed near the cabin and carried water back to make tea. After breakfast, while I was splitting some firewood, the dog returned. It jumped all over me, behaving like I was a long lost buddy. Apparently, any friend of Alonzo's was a friend of his.

II

One beautiful July morning Alonzo, his friend from Shubenacadie and I hiked to nearby Grand Lake to look for white ash which were plentiful there. He wanted the ash wood to make axe handles to sell to hardware stores in Halifax. We were walking in a hardwood stand near the lake when Alonzo showed me the segabun growing in a wet area. There were several of the plants in a small space. He dug up a bulb, examined it, then explained that it was good for chest ailments. He cut off a small piece of the bulb with his pocket knife and asked me to taste it. I should have suspected a trick because his friend had a silly grin on his face.

Foolishly, I chewed the segabun. At first it tasted somewhat like a potato. I fancied I liked it. Suddenly, I experienced a sharp pain in my mouth—it felt as if a knife had slit my tongue! It was awful. The pain lasted for a good minute before it subsided.

Alonzo laughed so hard at my predicament and peculiar facial expressions that he almost placed the lit end of a cigarette to his mouth. His friend, who thoroughly appreciated the joke, was resting against an old beech tree with tears of laughter in his eyes. I had learned about the segabun the hard way, and do not recommend the experience to anyone.[3] The plant contains crystals of oxalate of lime, which gives it the burning sensation. If it is allowed to dry for several months the crystals break down and the pungency disappears. It should be dried by cutting it in slices, as one would slice an onion.

Alonzo and his friend were apologetic and assured me I had passed their test. They said it was an old trick and that a lot of people had fallen victim to it, but few had expressed themselves as well as I had. We hiked to a stand of white ash, and Alonzo pointed out the trees which were best for making axe handles, baskets or other crafts. He explained that the grain must run straight and be free of knots. He said black ash was stronger but was much more difficult to find.

In the Autumn I returned to university for my final year. I was eager to begin my thesis on Micmac plant medicines. One day when I got back from the library there was a package waiting for me. It was post marked at Shubenacadie, loosely wrapped in brown paper, and tied with a string. I opened the package and found slices of segabun wrapped in newspaper. It was from Alonzo. He had remembered his promise from the summer and had sent slices of the segabun "not so sharp to the taste"!

Indian Turnip

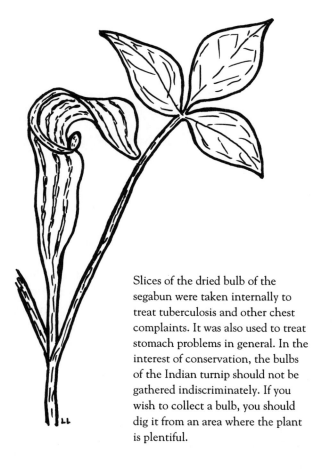

Slices of the dried bulb of the segabun were taken internally to treat tuberculosis and other chest complaints. It was also used to treat stomach problems in general. In the interest of conservation, the bulbs of the Indian turnip should not be gathered indiscriminately. If you wish to collect a bulb, you should dig it from an area where the plant is plentiful.

IN THE
PROTECTION OF
FRED'S COVE

Old Fred owned much of the woodland bordering the cove. He spent a good part of his life there cutting pulpwood and logs and hauling them to the roadside with his team of oxen. He died many years ago, but his name lives on. Fred's Cove forms part of the eastern shoreline of Minamkeak Lake. It is a short distance from my cabin if I cross through the medicine woods. At the far end of the cove are rows of weathered tree trunks, branches and root systems, known locally as "lakeshore wood." It is a reminder of when the town of Bridgewater built their dam on Minamkeak and flooded the area around the turn of the century.

There in an island in the cove where huckleberries grow in the hot days of July and August. In the winter it offers shelter from the cold northwest winds which blow over the frozen surface of Minamkeak. I have often taken refuge there to tie my skates. In the summer the cove is often calm when the lake is rough. It is possible

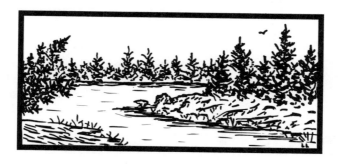

to see the flight of a bird reflected in the water. A canoe will remain still, resting against lily pads.

There are many species of trees near Fred's Cove. The stripped maple grows there, and I have seen the mountain ash, although that was a number of years ago. I found it while searching for medicine barks. It was growing on a small knoll overlooking the cove. There were a number of wild sarsaparilla plants nearby, and I think there was a raven's nest in the tall spruce trees which stand further back from the shore.

I have camped on the island where the huckleberries grow, and pitched my tent on a flat rock near the water's edge. The base of the tent was supported by rocks so that it would not collapse. The night was clear. A breeze from the northeast played with my camp fire, twisting and shaping the flames in a myriad of ways. I saw a fleeting image of an owl's wing where light met darkness over the water in front of me.

I woke to sounds outside my tent. There were footsteps on the rocks and the occasional splashing of water. Grabbing my flashlight, I gently lifted the tent flap, and stared into the darkness. I shone the light in several directions, but saw nothing. As I stepped outside, the tent collapsed! The rocks had been removed from the corners of the tent. In the mud I saw tracks of several raccoons, and a pan of beans which I had placed near the fire was licked clean. The raccoon is a trickster. The rocks were neatly piled to one side of the tent.

Lily
(Cow)

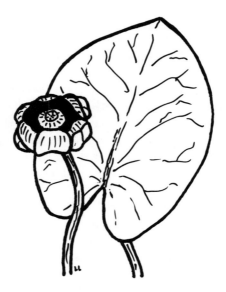

Cow lily was called "Big One Side" by the Micmac people. It was pounded into a mash and used to treat swollen limbs (Van Wart, p. 576, and personal notes recorded at Shubenacadie). The root was probably used for this purpose, although the leaves would also be effective medicinally.

Lily
(Water)

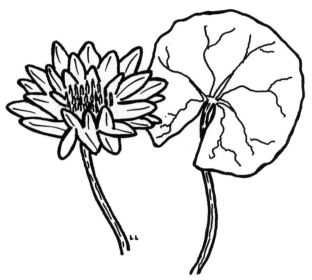

Water lily was used for the same purpose as that noted for the cow lily. The water in which the mashed root was boiled may be used as a bathing solution. Water lily root may have been steeped in water, and the liquid taken internally as a general preventive medicine. Some Micmac I spoke with implied that water lily root was *pagosi* ("bugosi"). If this is the case, it has very strong preventive medicinal qualities and may have been worn about the neck for this reason.

Maple

The bark of the white maple was
steeped in water until softened,
then applied to the chest as a
poultice to treat chest colds and
congestion. The stripped maple was
referred to as "moosewood" by the
Micmac. It may have been used to

Stripped Maple

treat swollen limbs (VanWart,
p. 576). The bark was used to make
a beverage (Wallis and Wallis,
p. 129). A person at Shubenacadie
told me about an incident which
apparently happened in the early
years of this century. He remarked,
"I know a man who worked on a
coal boat. This was in Saint John,
New Brunswick. The man had sore
eyes and he said can you help me? I
went and got some maple bark and
steeped it. He put this on his eyes.
Three weeks later I saw the man
and he told me that it cured his
eyes." I am uncertain of which type
of maple tree was used in the
treatment.

Mountain Ash

The bark of the mountain ash was
steeped in water and taken
internally to treat stomach pains.
Also, "round tree" was used to
counter a witch's bad wish (Wallis
and Wallis, p. 296).

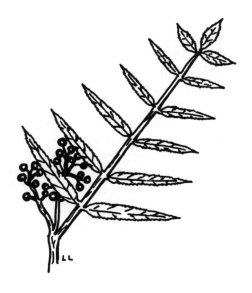

BURDOCK
AND OTHER
GOOD MEDICINES

A few years ago I participated in an oil painting workshop hosted by well-known Nova Scotia seascape artist, Graham "Buz" Baker. During the week-long workshop we made a painting excursion to Big Tancook Island off the coast of Chester, Nova Scotia. My job as an assistant was to help those people who were having problems with their paintings, especially the beginners in the class.

When the ferry docked at Big Tancook most of the people in our group immediately went off in search of scenes to paint and sketch. However, I was overwhelmed by something totally unrelated to painting or the workshop. The place was a mass of burdock! It was growing near the ferry dock, along the bank skirting the seashore and near the roadside. I remember swearing then and there that someday I would bring my brother's old bright red 1959 Chevrolet Apache half-ton to Tancook, and load it down to the axle with burdock. This never happened, but that day I did manage to fill my paint box with burdock roots.

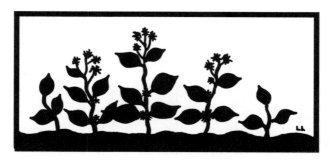

The burdock is one of my favourite medicinal plants; I have often felt tempted to plant a garden of it next to my cabin. It has been discussed extensively by many herbalists. As early as 1653 Nicolas Culpeper, in his *The English Physician*, extols the plant's effectiveness in treating skin disorders, bites, burns and kidney stones, among other ailments. He was probably referring to the *Arctium lappa L.* type which grows extensively in the British Isles.

The burdock was probably introduced into North America by the early European settlers. The Native people may have gained their knowledge of its medicinal qualities from those immigrants, who certainly would have been familiar with its medicinal uses. Burdock was used extensively as a medicinal plant by the Native people, and its many qualities are still widely recognized.

Witch grass was also introduced from Europe, and is considered both a curse and a blessing. I remember my father would complain angrily about witch grass because of the great difficulty he had in removing it from his garden. On the other hand, he valued the plant as a spring tonic. This is not surprising as the plant has a long history of usage as a general tonic.

Broad leaved plantain and yellow rattle are plants which occur throughout Nova Scotia, growing in lawns and fields, waste places and along the roadside. The plantain was introduced, although some botanists claim it may have been native to this province. The Micmac called it "white man's plantain" because it seemed to grow wherever white people settled, or to follow in their footsteps. Maud Grieve gives a similar explanation in her book, *A Modern Herbal*. She writes: "in both America and New Zealand it has been called by the aborigines the 'Englishman's Foot' (or the White Man's Foot), for wherever the English have taken possession of the soil, the Plantain springs up" (p. 36).

The yellow rattle is called "scared plant" because it makes a rattling noise when disturbed. A Micmac woman at Shubenacadie told me this during one of my visits there. She asked me if I had ever heard the rattling sound. I remarked that I had not, and that no one had mentioned or spoken about the scared plant. I followed her outside to the backyard, and as we walked through the grass she asked if I heard a popping sound. She said it was the yellow rattle. We were making the seed pods rattle as we walked amongst the plants. It is a delightful sound which I have experienced many times since that visit.

Myricaceas, the sweet gale family, is a group of spicy sweet scented plants found in abundance in the Maritime provinces. The sweet gale and bayberry belong in the genus *Myrica*, while the other member of the family, sweet fern, is of the genus *Comptonia*. The plants are useful as medicines, food flavourings and incense, and for removing obnoxious odours from pickle barrels or other containers.

The bayberry is plentiful near my cabin and can be found throughout the medicine woods. It likes to grow near the margin of lakes, swamps and bogs, and is usually abundant in old abandoned fields. Sweet fern grows in sandy and barren soils, and often occurs in large patches near highways and other open areas. The plant is referred to as "ant wood" as ants love to climb about on its branches. They are probably attracted by its delightful scent.

Other plants which grow near my cabin include the partridge-berry and teaberry or checkerberry. The teaberry is a wintergreen and grows in pastures, fields and barren land and in some cases is the primary ground cover of large areas. Its cousin, the snowberry or capillaire, is less prevalent and has white berries rather than the familiar red teaberry. The snowberry is found in moist mossy forests where conifers grow—the berries are delicious! Maud Grieve calls it "cancer wintergreen" because it is "supposed to remove the cancerous taint from the system" (pp. 849-50).

The partridgeberry occurs in mossy areas and is common throughout much of Nova Scotia. In Newfoundland people look forward to the partridgeberry season as they can be used in pies, jam and jelly. The type which grows in Nova Scotia is called "snakeberry" because the two eyes on the berry give it the appearance of a snake's head. The variety in Newfoundland has a single eye on its berry.

Bayberry

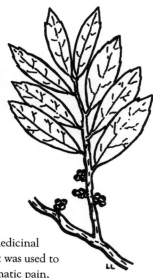

This berry has several medicinal
uses. The powdered root was used to
treat arthritic and rheumatic pain,
as were the leaves when used in
poultice form. The leaves and dried
roots, steeped in water, were taken
as a tea to treat mouth infections.
In this respect, the tea was used
regularly as a mouth wash.

Bunchberry

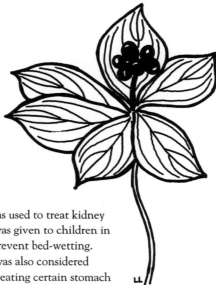

This plant was used to treat kidney ailments. It was given to children in tea form to prevent bed-wetting. Bunchberry was also considered effective in treating certain stomach problems, and the leaves were applied to wounds to stop bleeding and to promote healing. They were chewed and softened before being applied to the wound (Wallis, p. 26).

Burdock

The roots were used to treat and purify the blood. They were steeped in water and two or three cups of the beverage were taken daily. It is especially useful for treating skin disorders caused by impurities in the blood. A combination of burdock and red clover is considered an excellent blood tonic compound medicine by many herbalists.

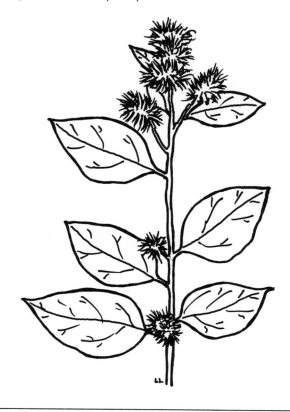

Buttercup

Arthur Van Wart writes that the Micmac used the buttercup to treat headaches and "pent-up feelings" (p. 576). The scent of the leaves or the juice from the leaves, applied to the nostrils, is said to cure headaches. The buttercup was also used to treat cancer. It would be placed over the diseased part of the body to "draw" the poison from the cancerous growth. The plant was probably softened by crushing and then applied in poultice form. There are several kinds of buttercups, some of which are probably stronger than others. The juice may cause blisters and, therefore, should be used with caution. They should *not be taken internally* unless skillfully combined with other herbs, and then *only under the supervision of a qualified herbalist.*

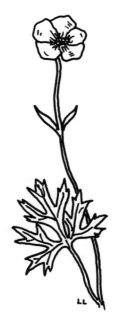

Clover
(Also, see burdock)

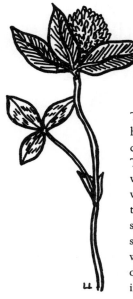

The Micmac used clover to treat high temperatures and feverish conditions (Van Wart, pp. 575-76). The plant was probably steeped in water and taken in tea form. A woman at Shubenacadie told me that clover was used to treat a bee sting. The juice was applied to the sting, or a plant poultice was used. I was unable to determine which kind of clover was most frequently used in these remedies.

Elder

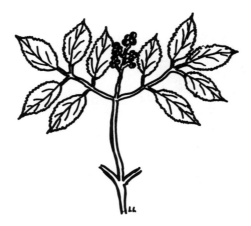

One source relates that the bark scraped upwards from the roots was used for emetic purposes. When scraped downwards it was used as a cathartic medicine. The plant was commonly called "pipe stem wood"[4] by the Micmac, and its leaves and bark may have been used as a tea (Van Wart, p. 574).

Indian Hemp

The plant was called "worm root" by the Micmac, and was used to expel worms. It was probably steeped in water and taken internally for this purpose (Van Wart, p. 573).

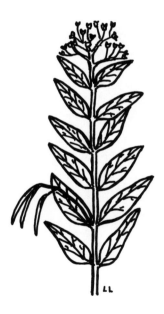

Meadow Beauty

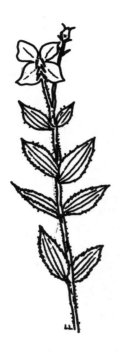

This plant is found growing in wet areas such as along lake shores. The Micmac may have used the meadow beauty as a wash to clean and clear the throat. The leaves and stem of the plant were steeped in water to produce a sour drink which was used for the above purpose.

Milkweed
(Common)

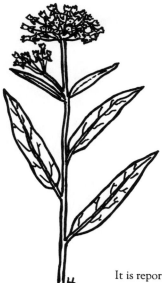

It is reported that this plant is effective in easing a poison ivy rash. The white juice from the milkweed is applied to the rash. I imagine swamp milkweed is also effective in this respect.

Pansy
(Field)

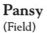

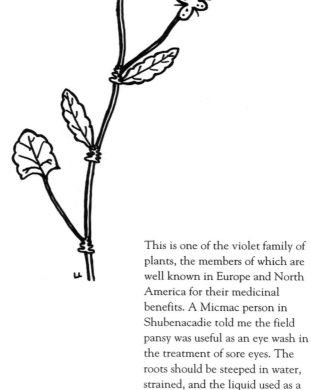

This is one of the violet family of plants, the members of which are well known in Europe and North America for their medicinal benefits. A Micmac person in Shubenacadie told me the field pansy was useful as an eye wash in the treatment of sore eyes. The roots should be steeped in water, strained, and the liquid used as a bathing solution.

Partridgeberry

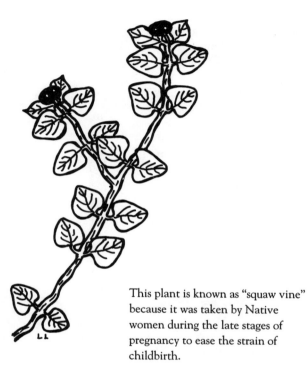

This plant is known as "squaw vine" because it was taken by Native women during the late stages of pregnancy to ease the strain of childbirth.

Plantain

The Micmac used plantain to draw poison from wounds and sores, and to effectively heal them. Apparently, they used the bark of the basswood tree for a similar purpose, that being to treat festering wounds. A woman from Eskasoni remarked that plantain can be used to treat stomach ulcers. She said the leaves should be steeped in water to produce a tea. It may be mixed with warm milk if desired.

Sweet Fern

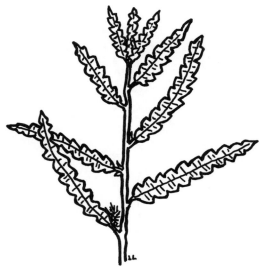

The sweet fern, like the milkweed, was used to treat poison ivy rash. The leaves would be steeped for a few minutes to soften them, then gently applied to the rash. I have never used the plant for this purpose, and have often wondered whether it is truly effective. Sweet fern was also used in poultice form as a treatment for rheumatism and external sores, and was steeped in water and used as a tea to be taken as a general tonic. I was told by a neighbour that he was cured of boils by a Micmac man who told him to steep the leaves and twigs of sweet fern in water. A tablespoon of the medicine was taken before each meal and before retiring for the night.

Teaberry

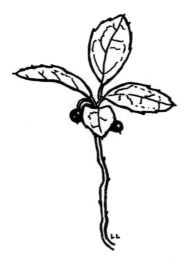

The Micmac probably had many uses for the teaberry plant. It is known as a preventive medicine against heart attacks, and as a medicine which can be used by a person recuperating from a heart attack. It is also useful for persons recovering from a stroke. The plant thins and regulates the blood, and in this manner aids circulation, preventing the formation of blood clots. To prepare the medicine, the entire plant should be steeped in water and the liquid used as a tea.

Waxberry

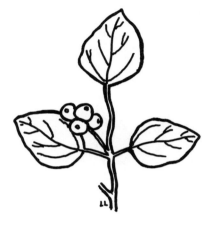

According to Wilson Wallis (p. 27), the Micmac used this plant to treat headaches. It would be tied into a bundle and sniffed for this purpose. A tonic was also made from the plant (Wallis and Wallis, p. 130). The waxberry is a member of the honeysuckle family; plants from this group are famous in European folk medicine as diuretics, purgatives and expectorants.

Witch Grass

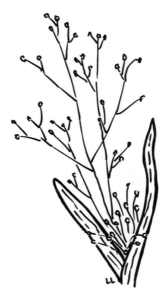

This was used as a general spring tonic to tune-up and invigorate the system. The grass was steeped in water and taken as a tea. I was told that it helped to revitalize the body "after a long hard winter."

Yarrow

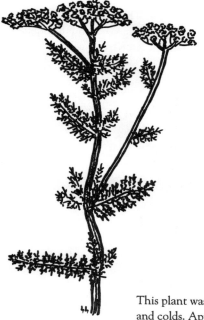

This plant was used to treat fevers and colds. Apparently, it induces perspiration when taken as a warm tea. Some people would allow it to steep in water for up to an hour, and then drink the tea mixed with warm milk. Yarrow stalks were also pounded into a pulp and applied to bruises, sprains and swellings. This was considered a very good treatment for those problems.

Yellow Rattle

This was used to treat "fits" and epilepsy. The entire plant should be steeped in water and the liquid taken internally.

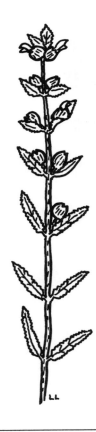

MEDICINAL
COMPOUNDS

A medicinal compound is a medicine composed of two or more active ingredients. For the most part, compound medicines used by the Micmac were combinations of plant and/or animal parts. They were often considered more potent than single medicinal potions because they utilized the combined power of a number of ingredients which worked together.

The preparation of medicinal compounds is an ancient practice, but early writings by explorers, missionaries and traders give little information on Micmac preparations. However, the rich compound medicine materials collected by Stansbury Hagar in the 1890s indicate that the Micmac had developed an extensive compound medicine tradition. There is evidence that some of this tradition survives today, given the information I was able to collect in Conne River, Newfoundland, concerning the "Seven Sorts" compound medicine (this is discussed in the Mystery Medicines chapter).

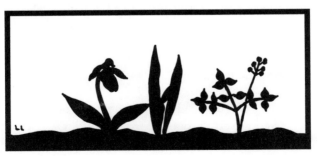

The medicinal compounds traditionally used by the Micmac were essentially of three types: edible and potable compounds, poultice compounds, and salve compounds (Lacey, pp. 38-40). During my research I collected a large number of compound remedies. Practically everyone I spoke with had a remedy or two they wished to share with me. I have listed below those which I feel will be of most interest to my readers.

■ ■ ■ ■

Compound Medicines

1. Black cherry and alder barks were steeped together in water, and the beverage taken as a **blood tonic**. I imagine that several cups of the tonic would be taken on a daily basis for a period of one to two weeks.

2. The sap of the balsam fir, mixed with black cherry bark and honey, was used to make a **cough syrup**. The black cherry bark was probably steeped in water, and a portion of the liquid added to the honey and balsam sap.

3. A combination of black cherry bark, balsam fir buds and ground juniper bark was steeped in water to produce a medicine effective in the treatment of **colds and influenza**.

4. The roots of wild sarsaparilla and sweet flag were crushed together and steeped in water to make a **cough medicine.**

5. Alder bark, boiled in water and mixed with porcupine fat, was used as a **cathartic medicine**.

6. A mixture of crushed plantain leaves and lamb's fat makes a salve effective in treating **sores**.

7.   A combination of spruce gum and lamb's fat was used to make a **salve**. The spruce gum was boiled in water. The coating which appeared on the surface of the water was removed and mixed with the lamb's fat.

8.   Blue violet plants were crushed and mixed with lamb's fat to produce a **salve** for general usage.

9.   The bark of the white pine was scraped and boiled in water until softened, and mixed with animal grease to produce a **salve**. It was used to heal wounds.

10.   Wild sarsaparilla root powdered and mixed with animal fat makes a **salve** for general usage.

11.   The bark of stripped maple and the bulb of the Indian turnip (well dried) were pounded and mixed together and steeped in water to produce a tea used to treat **colds**. The tea was sweetened with sugar or honey.

12.   A combination of hackmatack bark and skunk cabbage root was used to treat **tuberculosis**. The ingredients were probably steeped in water and the resulting medicine taken in small dosages.

MISCELLANEOUS FOLK REMEDIES

I

One has to learn to accept the unexpected in folk medicine as some remedies may appear ridiculous, and many downright harmful to the human constitution. Folk medicines must be recognized as expressions of efforts to confront illness and restore a sense of bodily well-being, otherwise the folklorist is apt to overlook and ignore things which were (are) very important to a community or cultural group.

A number of the remedies discussed in this section are common folk cures and are part of the traditional medicine practices of many peoples. The use of bear grease as a salve for external application is one such treatment, while goose grease was another very common salve. It was used by the Micmac to treat colds and congestion in the chest. Other remedies discussed herein are less common and some may be unique to Atlantic Canada or to the Micmac culture. For example, the fat of the owl was used as a salve or healing ointment

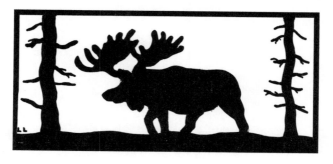

applied to treat aches and pains. It may have been rubbed on the chest to treat congestion. In some instances, fats from birds formed the basis for an ointment and herbal components were added to form the healing mixture. The "paunch" of an animal was used to treat those who had almost drowned. This may be uniquely Micmac, or a remedy confined to the Eastern Woodland peoples. Likewise, the use of sugar to treat "proud flesh" and eye disorders may be common in outport communities in Newfoundland, but not elsewhere.

There are folk remedies which have magical and/or ritual elements associated with their application and usage. Elsie Parsons writes of one such remedy which she collected from a Micmac woman in Cape Breton, Nova Scotia. It involved the use of spruce buds to cure warts. Parsons writes:

Take seven buds of the spruce tree and draw blood from one wart. Take one bud and dip it in the blood on the wart and then lay it on a piece of paper. Take another bud and dip in the same blood, but this time you rub it over another wart. Keep on doing this until you have rubbed all the warts and all the buds are on the paper. Enclose paper and buds in a parcel and leave it on the street until someone picks it up. Then your warts will go away. (p. 484)

In other remedies involving the treatment of warts, the materials are buried in the ground with the belief that the warts are buried with it. In this way, the person is cured. There is a psychological finality and transference expressed in the burying of the materials, and in their being carried away.

Another interesting remedy used a splinter taken from a tree which had been struck by lightning. Wallis and Wallis (p. 296) write that the splinter was used to cure toothaches. Apparently the lightning was thought to impart special qualities to the wood. They do not say how the cure was effected. I suspect that the splinter was considered a charm, and was carried on the person. It may have been carried in a pocket or perhaps sewn into a shirt collar or elsewhere on the clothing. This would not have been unusual as the Micmac used to do this with certain types of medicinal roots.

While toothaches were charmed away, earaches were often treated with tobacco smoke. The smoke was blown into the ear of the patient. Regular tobacco was used, or other varieties from that group of plants. In Native cultures several kinds of plants and tree barks were used as tobacco, either by themselves or combined in tobacco mixtures. Some of the mixtures were important both medicinally and in a religious and spiritual sense. Native people viewed life as one complete phenomenon and tended not to separate the spiritual from the physical, as is usually done in western society.

II

Poultices were used extensively in folk medicine. The mustard poultice was very popular and was a common remedy in Europe and North America. The Micmac used it to draw out the infection from wounds and sores of various kinds. A mustard bath was used to ease the pain of rheumatism. I spoke with a woman at Shubenacadie who told me that her cousin frequently bathed her feet in mustard water. This relieved the pain considerably and she was consequently able to walk without difficulty. But the relief is only temporary, so the process must be repeated. She said it can be made to last all day by sprinkling the dry mustard in one's stockings.

At Conne River several people mentioned the use of bread poultices as healing agents. One man told me the following story:

I helped a small baby and she is still living today. The child was ill so I went to get the nurse at St. Albans. When we returned from there the baby was just slumbering. The nurse, she just walked around the cot without even touching the baby. She said that it was too late to save the little girl. So, I took the nurse back to St. Albans and when I returned,

I stopped rowing, because I was sure I would hear the bell tolling for the girl. But when I got back she was still alive.

I told the women we should try to save the girl. One of the women asked, "What can we do? We'll do anything you tell us!" I told them to make a poultice out of soft bread, and to put it on the child. The next morning the girl was still alive in the cot, and she smiled at me as I walked past her.

I went again to fetch the nurse and she met me at the dock, and asked me how the baby was. I told her that the baby was better. The nurse asked me what I had done. I told her about the poultice. Well, we returned to the child, and the nurse tended to her until she finally recovered. I suppose the poultice helped her to recover.

Other stories at Conne River tell about the use of sugar for healing purposes. An elderly woman told me:

I had bad eyes, so I had to stay on a stool or chair because I could hardly see anything. One day I told my sister to open my eyes so I could put some sugar in them. Just a little sugar, because too much sugar will scratch the eyes! Then, I blinked my eyes in an ordinary way, and washed the sugar from my eyes with water. Well, I could see a little, so kept doing it and fixed my eyes quite a lot. Today, I can see as good as anyone. Sugar is good for cataracts. That's what ailed my eyes. I learned about using sugar for bad eyes by knowing that it will cure "proud flesh" by cutting it away from the hand.

There was a man from St. Albans who was blind. I told him that maybe I could help him, though it might be too late by now. I told him how sugar had cured my eyes. So, I mentioned what to do, but warned him not to blame me if he harms his eyes with too much sugar.

I never spoke to that man again. But I know that he's still in St. Albans. I don't know if he's blind yet or not; though, I notice that now he's able to walk along the road on his own.

Mustard, sugar and bread are just a few of the common household items which were used as healing agents in folk medicine. The list of items is long, and almost every one had a medicinal purpose. Kerosene, for example, was used to treat pneumonia. A cloth was soaked in it, then placed on the patient's chest. I told my mother about this remedy and she nodded in agreement. She commented that it was also used to treat toothaches and tonsillitis. For a toothache, kerosene was applied to the face; for tonsillitis the kerosene was applied to the throat. It was also used to treat a sore throat. For this purpose, a small amount of kerosene was added to sugar which the patient swallowed slowly. It was considered a very effective remedy. I asked her what she meant by "a small amount of kerosene" and she replied, "why just enough to dampen the sugar. It was a common thing in those days, because people didn't have money to have teeth pulled or to buy medicines."

III

Early Micmac society depended on securing an adequate supply of fish and game, especially during the harsh winter months. In this respect, the moose was probably more important than most animals as it provided food, clothing and even medicine. As regards the latter, Wilson and Ruth Wallis (p. 127) write that the moose contributed a substance which eased childbirth. They comment that there is a small bone, *oagando hi guidance* (found of the heart), which was "ground to powder, cooked in a broth and administered to the patient." Van Wart writes that the "bones of the legs and thighs of the moose after the marrow was eaten, were...reduced to a powder, the fragments were place in...boiling water, so that any remaining marrow or grease floated upon the surface of the boiling water" (p. 574). It was saved for later use. The soup was "white as milk" and was taken as a medicine, because it was "good for the chest."

Perhaps the earliest written account of the Micmac's medicinal uses of the moose is in Cretien LeClercq's *New Relations of Gaspesia*, published in 1691. He explains that "epilepsy was cured by using the left hind foot of a moose which had been seen to cure its epilepsy by scratching behind the ear with the same hoof" (p. 275). This is quite a remarkable remedy for epilepsy, and while we have no way of knowing the accuracy of LeClercq's description, it does show that the Micmac were close observers of the habits of animals. The extent of their knowledge of animal behaviour would no doubt astound us today.

An even more amazing remedy for those who have almost drowned was recorded by Sieur de Diereville in his manuscript of 1708:

> The Indians...cure themselves of death itself; what a paradox! it might be said, but I shall establish the fact. These wretched people are very liable to be drowned; it happens only too frequently, because their bark canoes capsize at the slightest provocation. Those who are fortunate enough to escape from the wreck make haste to rescue those who remain in the water. They then fill with tobacco smoke the bladder of some animal, or a long section of large bowel...and having tied one end securely, they fasten a piece of Pipe or Calumet into the other, to serve as an injection Tube; this is introduced into the backside of the Men who have drowned, and, by compressing it with their hands, they force into them the smoke contained in the bowel; they are afterwards tied by the feet to the nearest tree which can be found, and kept under observation; almost always follows the satisfaction of seeing that the smoke Douche forces them to disgorge all the water they have swallowed. Life is restored to their bodies, and before long this astonishing and beneficent result is made manifest by the twitching movements of the suspended Men. (p. 180)

The Micmacs' use of animal parts as medicines was in some respects as extensive and diverse as was their knowledge of plant remedies. For example, even mole's feet were used as a remedy. Wallis (p. 28) writes that they were placed on the body of a person as a temporary cure for convulsions. This type of remedy for seizures or convulsions is not unusual in folk medicine; people were willing to take extreme measures to combat ailments which appeared mysterious or incurable.

Other interesting remedies included using the contents of the gallbladder of an animal as a massage lubricant for rheumatic parts of the body. The urine from a porcupine bladder was used to treat earaches and defective hearing. It was dropped into the ear and retained there with a plug. The oil from the porcupine was given to children as a cathartic medicine. The meat itself was also taken as a medicine. A man in Eskasoni told me the following story:

At one time there was a smallpox epidemic in the village of...Barra Head. During the time of the epidemic, three men from the village decided to go away into the woods, probably to get away from the disease. Anyway, after they had gone about 50 miles...one of the men discovered he had the symptoms of the smallpox. So the other fellas built a shelter for the sick man, and got him some porcupine meat to eat. They even prepared and cooked the meat for him.

They left the sick man and continued on their journey. It was in the winter time so there wasn't any concern about the porcupine meat spoiling. In a while the men returned. As they approached the shelter, they figured they would find their friend dead of the smallpox. They called out his name and were surprised to hear him answer the call. He was still alive!

I imagine the porcupine meat was enough to keep him alive and to cure the smallpox. So, they got him fresh clothing to wear, burned the shelter, and returned to Barra Head.

Smallpox was introduced from Europe and ravaged Native populations in North America. In some instances, the disease was introduced deliberately by the Europeans in an effort to extermi-nate tribes. This amounted to a campaign of genocide against Native peoples who were not familiar with this disease and, conse-quently, were ill-prepared to combat it.

Other diseases, such as various types of measles, also presented grave problems for Native peoples, and for the general population. It resulted in the use of very innovative remedies. For instance, the Micmac used fresh droppings from deer to treat measles, and Natives and non-Natives alike used sheep manure for the same disease. Both the deer droppings and sheep manure were dissolved in water and taken internally. The idea was that the manure would force the measles "out on the skin," thus relieving the fever which accompanies the illness. These remedies reflect the desperate measures people took when confronted with terrible and unusual ailments and diseases.

IV

When I was a young boy, some years ago, I went fishing by a brook near Leipsigaek Lake. I came upon a still area of water surrounded by lush grasses and poplar trees. I thought I had found a secret fishing hole, so I prepared to cast my line to catch the big trout which I imagined to be there. What I had found was a beaver dam. It was at the far end of the pool. I tossed aside my little yellow rod, and hurried around the pool to examine how it was constructed. I saw teeth marks on various branches, and imagined watching the beaver carry them to the brook and place them in the dam.

In my teenage years I read Gray Owl's books, and could relate to his beaver people. His books, and my fascination with such discoveries as the beaver dam, were important experiences in my life. Those experiences are what the Buddhists call the "ordinary magic" of daily existence. They influence how we live the remainder of our lives.

The beaver, raccoon and skunk were used for medicinal purposes. A woman at Conne River told me that the contents of the gallbladder of a beaver is a remedy for "stones" if taken internally. A second person claimed that "beaver castors, the two things back there by the beaver's pelvis," (the sex glands) make a good medicine, but did not give specific uses. He was more familiar with the raccoon. He told me that its oil is a good cathartic medicine for children, while the grease from the animal is useful for treating rheumatism. It should be rubbed on the flesh for this purpose.

Skunk oil is a well known folk remedy. It was toted as a cure for baldness, and was promoted in this fashion by the travelling medicine shows. The oil was rubbed on the scalp and was supposed to rejuvenate hair roots. I spoke with a woman in Shubenacadie who was convinced that skunk oil would indeed promote hair growth. She said that it was also useful for treating rheumatism, and for relieving colds, feverish conditions and earaches. The oil was dropped into the ear to treat the latter. This remedy was used in many parts of North America.

There are other common folk cures which are well-known in Micmac culture. For instance, eel skin was used to treat lameness. The "slimy" side of the skin was applied to the lame area of the body. It was also a cure for headaches. In this case the skin was tied around the head of the patient. It was applied to the body to treat cramps and rheumatism, or fitted tightly against the flesh to treat sprains. It is interesting to note that snake skin was used for similar purposes. The shed skin of a snake was said to cure a headache when tied around the head of a patient. This was reported by Wallis in 1922 (p. 27). He also observed that the dried tongue of a snake was a charm, especially effective in curing toothaches.

There was an elderly woman in Conne River who was well known for her ability to charm teeth. This person was capable of "absent" charming; that is, curing toothaches from a distance, without physical contact with the patient. People in the neighbouring community of St. Albans would often use her services. They would explain the problem over the telephone, and the woman would produce a cure shortly afterwards. She is said to have received her charm from the Christian Bible. People at Conne River say that a local anaesthesia will not relieve the pain of a charmed tooth. However, when the charming takes effect, the ache will not return. Later, the tooth will fall out.

MYSTERY
MEDICINES

In the 1890s an American folklorist, Stansbury Hagar, visited Nova Scotia to do research on Micmac culture. He visited the Digby area of the province and may have gone elsewhere. In 1896 he published an article based on material collected during his sojourn in Nova Scotia in the *Journal of American Folk-Lore*. I wish I had been around in the 1890s when Hagar was doing his research. There is something about the man which is intriguing and, from a folklore perspective, his work is important because he gives us a glimpse into Micmac culture which is not otherwise available, and which is probably lost today.

In his "Micmac Magic and Medicine," Hagar writes about magical herbs. He notes that there is a plant which the Micmac call *mededeskooi*, the "rattling plant." The plant has three leaves which produce the sound of the rattlesnake when they rub together. It stands about knee high, with leaves about eight inches long and

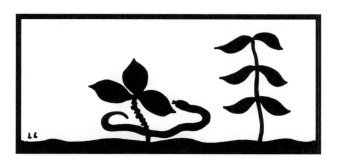

shaped like those of the poplar. The root is the size of one's fist, and the stalk is surrounded with numerous brownish-yellow balls the size of buckshot. Apparently, the Micmac described the plant as resembling the wild turnip. They must have meant the segabun, or Indian turnip.

Hagar met only one person who claimed to have seen the plant, and observed that generally the Micmac were reluctant to talk about the mededeskooi. Stephen Bartlett, who claimed to have seen it, described the plant as smaller than he had expected. When he returned the following morning, the plant had disappeared. This is because he had neglected to perform the proper ceremony, or to approach the plant in the correct manner.

In his description, Hagar explains that you must follow the cooasoonech (a bird dwelling in old logs) who will take you to the plant. Otherwise, it is invisible. When the bird sings, follow it, until eventually you will hear the rattling leaves of the magic plant. Shortly afterwards the plant will appear. Then, you must gather thirty sticks and lay them in a pile near the plant, before leaving that place. When you return, you must be with a girl, the more beautiful the better, and both must approach the plant crawling on hands and knees. It is inhabited by the spirit of a rattlesnake, which will come forth and circle the plant. You must pick up the snake, which will then disappear. Hagar completes his description, by writing:

The plant must be divided into four portions…three may be taken…one must be left standing. The three parts are scraped and steeped and a portion wore about the person. Some say that, divided in seven parts, this medicine will cure seven diseases, but the great majority believe that it will cure any disease and gratify any wish. It is held to be especially potent as a love-compeller. (pp.176-77)

The reference to the rattlesnake is interesting in light of the fact that this snake does not live in the eastern part of the continent.

Also, Hagar's comment that the medicine can be worn "about the person" to prevent illness, is characteristic of several other Micmac medicines, such as the flagroot, segabun and pagosi.

Wilson and Ruth Wallis, in their ethnography of the Micmac, mention a plant similar in some respects to the mededeskooi.

Another good medicine…is a tall plant which has six leaves, in pairs, one pair directly over the other. Some men who found it blazed a tree alongside it, so that they could find it later. When they returned to get it they…could not find it. I myself, in company with some others, found one. We left our axes by it, and went to dinner. When we returned…it was gone. An old woman once told me, "you must put a penny on the ground, over the roots; the plant will then not go away." In the old days people placed the kneecap of an animal over its roots, and the plant would then not go away.

If you drink tea made from it and rub some of the plant on your hands and face, you can sleep next to a person with smallpox or anything else, and you will not contact the disease. (p. 129)

There must have been a rich genre of such plant legends which are now lost to the culture.

Stansbury Hagar also discusses a special compound medicine made from seven ingredients: alum bark, hornbeam bark, beech bark, wild willow bark, wild blackberry bark, ground hemlock root and red spruce root. They must be gathered in the autumn and in the order given above. He describes how to collect the barks and roots, and mentions that the compound is used for both internal and external purposes.

The trunk of every tree is divided into four sections supposed to face the sun between sunrise, at dawn, noon, sunset, and midnight. In the forenoon one should cut the bark from the direction of sunrise as far as the direction of the sun at noon, but no further. This is the most propitious quarter, hence medicine gathered from it will yield the best results. In the afternoon cut from the noon point to the sunset point. This quarter is propitious, though less so. Bark gathered from the other two quarters or from the right quarter at the wrong time is at least useless, often poisonous. For the sunlight purifies the side it touches, but the shadow is hostile to life. The roots should extend from the trunk towards the propitious side. (p. 174)

In Conne River I met a person who taught me how to collect and prepare a similar compound medicine. It is called the Seven Sorts medicine, and was considered a panacea by many of the elderly residents. In fact, people of all age groups were familiar with the medicine, and there were numerous accounts of its healing powers. However, very few people seemed to know the contents of the medicine and how to prepare it. Those who spoke about its contents remarked that some of the ingredients can vary, while others remain constant. The final nature of the medicine depended on who was preparing it.

The medicine is made from equal amounts of the bark of poplar, hackmatack, dogwood, bird or pin cherry,[5] pussy willow and ground juniper. These are combined with a proportion of gold thread approximately equal in strength to each of the other ingredients. The mixture is then steeped or boiled in water depending on whether it is to be used for internal or external purposes. For internal use, the medicine is steeped and the liquid taken in beverage form. For external use, the mixture is boiled until a black, molasses-like state is achieved. The medicine is applied in poultice or plaster form to the injured area of the body. In the past, it was spread on brown paper and applied in that fashion.

The Seven Sorts compound was used to treat most ailments. When applied as a poultice it will help to mend broken bones, treat bruises, cure a lame back and heal skin cancer. The poultice or plaster is supposed to move during the curative process. I was told that during the course of the treatment, the pain of an ailment will tend to move from the body in a particular direction. The poultice will move in the direction the pain takes as it leaves the body. When the pain disappears, and a cure is effected, the poultice will fall from the body.

During a visit to Eskasoni I discovered that the pussy willow, in poultice form, is said to move over the body in a manner similar to the Seven Sorts medicine. It is also boiled to a molasses-like state, and is considered useful in treating most ailments. However, the Micmac I spoke with in Eskasoni, were not familiar with the Seven Sorts compound. Yet, the instructions for preparing the pussy willow medicine, and its uses, were identical to those described for the Seven Sorts medicine.

The ingredients comprising the Seven Sorts medicine are different from those listed by Stansbury Hagar for his compound preparation. However, I believe the Micmac were aware of the Seven Sorts preparation, even in Hagar's day. In his article, Hagar remarks: "the most powerful of all known in Micmac *materia medica* [is]...a mixture of seven such compounds as the one just described. It therefore contains forty-nine ingredients" (p. 174). I like to think that the Seven Sorts medicine is one of those seven compounds, or a variation thereof.

PREPARATION INSTRUCTIONS FOR SOME COMMON MEDICINAL TEAS

Alder
One ounce* of bark to one pint** of water. Bring water to the boil, then allow to steep for ten minutes. Take one-half to one cup to treat stomach cramps.

Bearberry
One ounce of dried leaves to one pint of water. Bring to boil and allow to steep for twenty minutes. Take one cup of the tea daily for general tonic purposes.

Beech
One ounce of leaves to one and a half pints of water. Bring water to boil and steep for fifteen minutes. Take one cup twice daily for general tonic purposes.

Birch (Yellow)
One ounce of inner bark to one pint of water. Bring to boil and steep for ten minutes. Take one cup of the tea to relieve cramps and diarrhoea.

Blackberry
One ounce of bruised root, bark or leaves to one and a half pints of water. Bring water to a boil and steep for twenty minutes. Drink one half to a cup of the tea to relieve diarrhoea and the effects of "summer sickness."

Boneset

One ounce to one and a half pints of water. Bring water to a boil and steep for ten minutes. Take half a cup twice daily for general tonic purposes.

Burdock

One ounce of dried root to one and a half pints of water, and allow to boil down to one pint of water. Take two cups of the tea daily for general tonic purposes.

Clover (Red)

One ounce of the dried plant to one pint of water. Bring water to a boil and steep for ten minutes. Take one cup of the tea daily for general tonic purposes.

Fir (Balsam)

One ounce of the bark and twigs steeped in one pint of water for fifteen minutes produces a tea pleasing to the taste, and useful in treating colds. Take two to three cups daily.

Gold Thread

Add twelve inches of gold thread to two cups of water. Bring water to a boil and allow to steep for fifteen minutes. This is excellent for promoting an appetite. Drink one half cup of the tea twice daily.

Labrador Tea

One ounce of leaves to one and a half pints of water. Bring water to a boil and steep for ten minutes. This makes a pleasing tonic tea for occasional usage.

Pine(White)

One ounce of bark, needles or twigs to one and a half pints of water. Bring to a boil and steep for ten minutes. Take two cups daily to treat colds.

Raspberry
The same as for the blackberry tea above.

Spruce (Black)
The same as for the fir tea above.

Strawberry
Six teaspoons of fresh or dried leaves to one pint of boiling water. Allow to steep for fifteen minutes. Take one cup of the tea two to three times daily. This is excellent for stomach cramps and for dysentery.

Teaberry
Fill a quart jar to the top with freshly picked leaves, then fill the jar with boiling water. Allow covered jar to stand in a warm place for a couple of days. Prepare to serve by heating the contents (Gibbons, p. 92). This makes a pleasing tea for occasional usage. It was used as a blood thinner to combat blood clotting.

Wild Sarsaparilla
Use one half ounce of the powdered root to one pint of water. Bring to a boil and steep for fifteen minutes. Take one half cup of the medicine three times daily for colds and influenza.

Yarrow
Use one ounce of the dried plant to one pint of water. Bring water to a boil and allow to steep for fifteen minutes. Take a cup of the tea twice daily to relieve fever and colds.

*1 ounce = 28.350 grams   **1 pint = 0.473 litres

ENDNOTES

1   I highly recommend Roland and Smith's *The Flora of Nova Scotia*. It is my plant bible and favourite manual. The book has good descriptive notes on the characteristics of plants, and specifies where they are found in the province. It contains maps and excellent illustrations.

2   The question of when to gather medicine barks and plant materials deserves some comment. Several of my Native sources believed that generally medicines should be collected in the late summer or early autumn. This is when plant life has fully matured and has not yet begun breaking down to complete its cycle. There are exceptions, of course, like the skunk cabbage root, which must be collected very early in the summer before the plant rots away. If one wishes to collect blossoms for tea or medicines, the time for collecting may vary greatly between plants. Barks may be collected year-round, although from some trees it might be more potent in late summer or early autumn. A couple of my sources would not collect medicines unless they were required at the moment. They believed regardless of the season, there was always a medicine available in nature for the ailment.

Overall, if someone wishes to collect medicines and teas, the late summer is fine for a large number of plants. However, you may want to watch each plant individually, note when it matures, and collect material shortly afterwards.

3   I do not recommend playing this "old trick" on anyone. The fresh bulb of the Indian turnip may cause swelling in the throat area, leading to breathing difficulties. It could result in death.

4   In this regard see *Rand's Micmac Dictionary*. Both Wallis (p. 24) and Van Wart (p. 576) suggests that "pipe stem wood" is the alder tree. I believe that elder is the correct designation, not only because of what Rand says but, also, because it has a hollow centre.

5   In the Seven Sorts preparation, black cherry bark may be used as a substitute for the pin cherry bark. The inner bark of the cherry is used in the medicine.

BIBLIOGRAPHY

Anonymous. "Micmac Medicine," *Micmac News*, vol. 4, no. 9 (1974).

Clark, Jeremiah S. *Rand's Micmac Dictionary*. Charlottetown: The Patriot Publishing, 1902.

Diereville, Sieur de. *Relations of the Voyage to Port Royal in Acadia or New France*. Toronto: The Champlain Society, 1933. (Originally published in 1708.)

Gibbons, Euell. *Stalking the Healthful Herbs*. New York: David MacKay Company Ltd., 1975.

Grieve, Maud. *A Modern Herbal*. Middlesex: A Peregrine Book, Penguin Books, 1976. (Originally published in 1931.)

Hagar, Stansbury. "Micmac Magic and Medicine," *Journal of American Folklore*, vol. 9 (1896).

Lacey, Laurie. *Micmac Indian Medicine: A Traditional Way of Health*. Antigonish, Nova Scotia: Formac Publishing, 1977.

LeClercq, Cretien. *New Relations of Gaspesia with the Customs and Religion of the Gaspesian Indians*. Toronto: The Champlain Society, 1910. (Originally published in 1691.)

Parsons, Elsie Clews. "Micmac Notes," *Journal of American Folk-lore*, vol. 39 (1926).

Roland, A.E. and E.C. Smith. *The Flora of Nova Scotia*. Halifax: The Nova Scotia Museum, 1969.

Van Wart, Arthur. "The Indians of the Maritime Provinces, their Diseases and Native Cures," *Canadian Medical Association Journal*, vol. 59 (1948).

Wallis, Wilson. "Medicines Used by the Micmac Indians," *American Anthropologist*, vol. 24 (1922).

Wallis, Wilson and Ruth Wallis. *The Micmac Indians of Eastern Canada*. Minnasota: The University of Minnasota Press, 1955.

PLANT INDEX

Standard Name	Latin Name	Pages
Alder	*Alnus crispa* (Ait.) Pursh, *Alnus rugosa* (DuRoi) Spreng., and most other types 20, 22, 30, 98, 114, 118	
Ash (white)	*Fraxinus americana* L. 1, 67, 68	
Bayberry	*Myrica pensylvanica* L. 78, 79	
Bearberry	*Anctostaphylos Uva-ursi* (L.) Spreng. 32, 114	
Beech	*Fagus grandifolia* Ehrh 2, 31, 46, 47, 50, 68, 111, 114	
Birch (Yellow)	*Betula allegheniensis* Britt. 2, 31, 47, 51, 114	
Blackberry	*Rubus allegheniensis* Porter, *Rubus canadensis* L. and other varieties .... ix, 40, 42, 111, 114	
Bloodroot	*Sanguinaria canadensis* L. 2, 6	
Blue Flag	*Iris versicolor* L. ....x, 23	
Blue Violet	*Viola cucullata* Ait. 99	
Blueberry	*Vaccinium myrtilloides* Michx. ..40, 41, 43	
Boneset	*Eupatorium perfoliatum* L. 31, 33, 115	
Bunchberry	*Cornus canadensis* L. 80	

Standard Name	Latin Name	Pages
Gold Thread	*Coptis trifolia* L.	61, 63, 67, 112, 115
Hackmatack	*Larix laricina* (DuRoi) K. Koch.	36, 48, 49, 55, 99, 112
Hemlock	*Tsuga canadensis* (L.) Carr.	56, 111
Horse Radish	*Amoracia rusticana* (Lam.) G.M. and S.	3, 10
Huckleberry	*Gaylussacia baccata* (Wang.) K. Koch.	70, 71
Indian Hemp	*Apocynum cannabinum* L.	85
Indian Tobacco	*Lobelia inflata* L.	2, 3, 11
Indian Turnip	*Arisaema Stewardsonii* Britt.	4, 66, 69, 99, 110, 111, 118
Juniper (Common)	*Juniperus communis* L.	34, 98, 112
Labrador Tea	*Ledum groenlandicum* Oeder.	3, 12, 115
Lady's Slipper	*Cypripedium acaule* Aito., and other varieties	13
Lambkill	*Kalmia augustifolia* L.	14
Lily (Cow)	*Nuphar variegatum* Engelm.	72
Lily (Water)	*Nymphaea odorata* Ait.	73
Maple	*Acer pensylvanicum* L. and probably *Acer saccharum* Marsh. and other species	2, 71, 74, 99
Meadow Beauty	*Rhexia virginica* L.	86

Standard Name	Latin Name	Pages
Milkweed (Common)	*Asclepias syriaca* L. and probably *A. incarnata* L.	87, 91
Mountain Ash	*Sorbus americana* Marsh.	71, 75
Mullein (Common)	*Verbascum virgatum* Stokes.	30, 31, 35
Oaks	*Quercus* L.	48, 57
Pansy (Field)	*Viola arvensis* Murr.	88
Partridgeberry	*Mitchella repens* L.	78, 89
Pine (White)	*Pinus Strobus* L.	29, 36, 99, 115
Pitcher Plant	*Sarracenia purpurea* L.	26
Plantain	*Plantago major* L.	77, 90, 98
Poison Ivy	*Rhus radicans* L.	30
Poplar	*Populus* L. (several varieties)	37, 107, 112
Prince's Pine	*Chimaphila umbellata* (L.) Bart.	2, 15
Pussy Willow	*Salix discolor* Muhl. and other varieties	18, 112, 113
Raspberry	*Rubus strigosus* Michx., and other varieties	40, 44, 116
Skunk Cabbage	*Symplocarpus foetidus* (L.) a Nutt.	4, 16, 99, 117
Snowberry	*Gaultheria hispidula* (L.) Muhl.	78
Sphagnum Moss	*Sphagnum palustre* L.	62
Spruce	*Picea* Dietr. (serveral varieties)	38, 60, 62, 71, 99, 101, 111, 116